PUBLIC HEALTH IN THE 21ST CENTURY

# BEAUTY AND HEALTH

# PUBLIC HEALTH
# IN THE 21ST CENTURY

PUBLIC HEALTH IN THE 21ST CENTURY

# BEAUTY AND HEALTH

## ZENOBIA C. Y. CHAN

### EDITOR

**Nova Science Publishers, Inc.**

*New York*

For permission to use material from this book please contact us:
Telephone 631-231-7269; Fax 631-231-8175
Web Site: http://www.novapublishers.com

## NOTICE TO THE READER

The Publisher has taken reasonable care in the preparation of this book, but makes no expressed or implied warranty of any kind and assumes no responsibility for any errors or omissions. No liability is assumed for incidental or consequential damages in connection with or arising out of information contained in this book. The Publisher shall not be liable for any special, consequential, or exemplary damages resulting, in whole or in part, from the readers' use of, or reliance upon, this material. Any parts of this book based on government reports are so indicated and copyright is claimed for those parts to the extent applicable to compilations of such works.

Independent verification should be sought for any data, advice or recommendations contained in this book. In addition, no responsibility is assumed by the publisher for any injury and/or damage to persons or property arising from any methods, products, instructions, ideas or otherwise contained in this publication.

This publication is designed to provide accurate and authoritative information with regard to the subject matter covered herein. It is sold with the clear understanding that the Publisher is not engaged in rendering legal or any other professional services. If legal or any other expert assistance is required, the services of a competent person should be sought. FROM A DECLARATION OF PARTICIPANTS JOINTLY ADOPTED BY A COMMITTEE OF THE AMERICAN BAR ASSOCIATION AND A COMMITTEE OF PUBLISHERS.

Additional color graphics may be available in the e-book version of this book.

LIBRARY OF CONGRESS CATALOGING-IN-PUBLICATION DATA

Chan, Zenobia C. Y.
  Beauty and health / Zenobia C. Y. Chan, Queeni T.Y. Ip.
     p. ; cm.
  Includes bibliographical references and index.
  ISBN 978-1-61209-832-6 (softcover)
  1. Surgery, Plastic--China--Hong Kong. 2. Health. I. Ip, Queeni T. Y.
II. Title.
  [DNLM: 1. Surgery, Plastic--Hong Kong. 2. Cosmetic Techniques--Hong
Kong. WO 600]   RD118.C42 2011     617.9'5--dc22
                                                           2011002413

*Published by Nova Science Publishers, Inc.* ✦ *New York*

# CONTENTS

# PREFACE

There are no cosmetic surgery (CS) statistics available in Hong Kong. CS has become popular and common in Hong Kong, especially with the emergence of beauty salons to which clients have easy access. However, there was found to be too little support for those undergoing and becoming addicted to CS, and whose health is affected as a result. Eyelash beauty treatments are assumed to improve ethnic "deficiencies" and bring psychological benefits in terms of femininity, normalcy, and self-management. Frequent treatments and chemical products place stress on the eye and are closely related to a person's health in general. Eyebrow beauty treatments are commonly available in Hong Kong salons and elsewhere. Nail care should be seen as personal hygiene, but beautiful nails are perceived as a representation of feminine beauty. Recently, artificial fingernails have become very popular in Hong Kong. A lack of literature about nail beauty and women's health in Hong Kong and elsewhere has been found. Microneedle therapy or skin needling can remove the lipids from cells and increase the hydrophilic molecule diffusion rate coefficient. Hence the anti-ageing approach can be reached. Certainly there are other benefits resulted from microneedle therapy. There are no literature regarding stem-cell cosmetics and health has been published in Hong Kong. Many unexplored rooms and hidden risks of this therapy should be studied. Although stem-cell cosmetics therapy can raise the quality of life in the coming dominated elderly population, health prevention and education should promote the unbiased appraisal of stem-cell cosmetics at the same time for public before taking action. Anti-aging should be a preventative health care topic in the coming future because of the growing elderly population.

# Chapter 1

# COSMETIC SURGERY RESEARCH

## *Zenobia C. Y. Chan and Queeni T. Y. Ip*

The Hong Kong Polytechnic University, China

## ABSTRACT

A cross sectional study is objected to examine the personal, social and perceptional factors of cosmetic surgery (CS) for women in Hong Kong. 162 Hong Kong women from November 2009 to January 2010 were recruited. A hundred female candidates completed a self-report questionnaire that assessed CS in Hong Kong by snowball sampling. Personal, social and perceptional information were then collected to estimate the risk factors of CS use and addiction. Personal factors including age ($p=0.000$), income ($p=0.000$) and education ($p=0.000$), social factors such as family ($p=0.001$), media ($p=0.004$), atmosphere ($p=0.018$) and acceptance ($p=0.000$), and objection ($p=0.023$) were all positively associated with CS and addiction. It is concluded that risk factors for CS addiction are indicated, which are crucial in offering insights for health education and health promotion on CS with a view to preventing addiction.

# INTRODUCTION

There should be plastic but not cosmetic surgery in Hong Kong. Plastic surgery includes reconstructive surgery and aesthetic surgery, which are performed by specialists in plastic surgery (Hong Kong Society of Plastic, Reconstructive and Aesthetic Surgeons, 2008) who are approved by the Hong Kong Academy of Medicine, HKAM. However, many CS services provided by beauty salons or medical beauty centers (to be generally called cosmetic surgery centers, CSC, below) which are not monitored in Hong Kong. Their experience, trust, and techniques are different. Finally, beauty accidents and complaints will result (Consumer Council, 2007 & 2008).

Customers can easily access CS in CSCs, and the trend of seeking CS is increasing in both mainland China (Watts, 2004) and Hong Kong (Lok, 2007). Former Miss Hong Kong Natalie Ng Man-yan is the first "artificial" actress and a proponent of "cosmetic tours" to Korea, having had CS herself in 2007 (Lok, 2007). Also, the trend is increasing across different age groups (China News, 2008). A ten-year-old girl was afraid of bullying from her classmates and thus urged her mother to accept her double eyelid surgery (The Sun, 2010). People are very accepting because of the growth of surgical techniques and idol presentation (The Sun, 2010).

However, two possible problems directly affecting public health may emerge. First, CS accidents or complaints will increase if CS remains unclear and without any legislation or monitoring. Second, CS addiction will be another problematic issue after drug addiction.

No literature has addressed the issue of CS addiction in Hong Kong. Therefore, this study will explore CS in Hong Kong and aims to enhance the professionalism of related industries by analyzing the existing Hong Kong CS situation, identifying the patients at most risk of becoming beauty junkies, and referring them to in-depth counseling before undergoing surgery to prevent addiction. CS is a hot trend in the medical and beauty fields in Hong Kong (HKACCS, 2007). We foresee that it will be considered part of caring services in the future. This pilot study hopes to give a fundamental understanding of this area to nurses and practitioners.

It was concluded that CS is generally portrayed as a risky but worthwhile option for women to enhance both their physical appearance and emotional health (Polonijo & Carpiano, 2008). Blum (2005) has described the culture of CS. Predictors of young women's interest in obtaining CS were also examined in the Northeastern United States and all were correlated with women's interest in CS (Markey & Markey, 2009). However, no similar studies have been found in Hong Kong.

There has been literature discussing plastic or aesthetic surgery in Hong Kong, but none dealing with CS. Literature about CS addiction is very general, but not in Hong Kong. CS in Hong Kong is now debatable in the city but no literature illustrating the CS and addiction of Hong Kong women has been found. Furthermore, there is no literature about the health risks of CS and prevention of CS addiction. Hence, this study will explore more about the CS of Hong Kong women as females dominate the beauty salons (Hong Kong Trade Development Council, 2001) and give insight to health promotion and education.

We found risks for CS. First, patients often seek the advice of beauticians, family and friends before going to a licensed medical professional for skin treatment (Karnani, 2007). Second, the definition of aesthetic surgery is not clear in Hong Kong. Third, surgeries are not required to be performed by specialists in plastic surgery (Consumer Council, 2008). Fourth, the differences between medical beauty services and CS services are unclear (Consumer Council, 2008). That is why members of the specialty have to accept some of the blame for the misunderstanding and misconceptions surrounding what they do (Kumar et al., 2007). Fifth, misleading advertisements or trade descriptions of services like non-surgical cosmetic treatments can mislead customers into having CS (Consumer Council, 2007). Sixth, both cosmetic and aesthetic surgery can easily cause physical and psychological dependence which produce pleasure and provide an escape from internal discomfort (Goodman, 2006). The above confusion, misleading information, and dependence definitely confirm the importance of knowledge of CS and addiction. We urge health promotion and education on CS. This study aims to fill this knowledge gap in Hong Kong.

## Definitions of Key Terms of this Study

"CS" is performed to reshape the normal structures of the body in order to improve the patient's appearance and self-esteem. "Hong Kong Women" are females of all ages who are Chinese and have lived in Hong Kong over seven years. "Addiction" denotes a process whereby a behavior can function to produce pleasure and is characterized by recurrent failure to control the behavior and continuation of the behavior despite significant negative consequences (Goodman, 2006).

# METHODS

## Study Population and Field Methods

We recruited 162 Hong Kong women from November 2009 to January 2010 as 12% prevalence resulted in previous study (YWCA, 2004). We used a snowball sampling strategy to respect the sensitivity and privacy of Hong Kong women. Data on personal, social and perceptional factors were collected via electronic anonymous self-administered surveys that were sent to one woman known to be working in the beauty sector by email at the beginning of the study. The response rate was 62%. The study protocol was approved by the Ethics Committee of the Hong Kong Polytechnic University.

## Data Analyses

Between January and February 2010, we calculated categorical and dichotomous predictors by Chi-square test in order to test the correlation between surgery and the outcome variables. The categorical variables considered as predictors were the women's age (year<18, 18-29, 30-50 or >50), marital status (single, married or divorced), income (<HK$10K, $10K-19.999K, $20K-30K or >$30K), education (secondary, tertiary, or postgraduate level), and indicators of the CSC, including beauty center, medical beauty center or aesthetic surgery center. The remaining dichotomous outcomes included doctor, family, media, atmosphere, acceptance, safety, injection, happiness, permanency, objection, reason and future. We then obtained the prevalence for each outcome and statistical significance at the $p<0.05$ level. Next, we tested for magnitude in the factors of CS and addiction by categorical and dichotomous variables using the Kendall tau-b and McNemar tests, respectively. We obtained the value and retained variables that were statistically significant at the $p<0.05$ level. We conducted all analyses using the SPSS software version 15.0.

**Table 1. Cosmetic surgery study of women from Hong Kong**

| | Cosmetic Surgery in Hong Kong n=100 | | | | | |
|---|---|---|---|---|---|---|
| Personal | Prevalence[a] (%) | | | | Correlates of cosmetic surgery (p) | Correlates of cosmetic surgery addiction (value,p) |
| Age, years | <18 | 18-29 | 30-50 | >50 | 0.038 | 0.385, 0.000 |
| | 4 | 50 | 44 | 2 | | |
| Marital Status | Single | Married | Divorced | | 0.253 | - |
| | 77 | 22 | 1 | | | |
| Income, HK$ | <$10k | $10k-19,999 | $20k-30k | >$30k | 0.000 | 0.359, 0.000 |
| | 19 | 40 | 25 | 16 | | |
| Education Level | Secon-dary | Tertiary | Post-gra-duate | | 0.030 | 0.398, 0.000 |
| | 17 | 54 | 29 | | | |
| Social | Yes | No | | | | |
| Encouraged by family | 20 | 80 | | | 0.000 | 0.733, 0.001 |

**Table 1. Continued**

| Attracted by media | 37 | 63 | | | 0.001 | 0.478, 0.004 |
|---|---|---|---|---|---|---|
| CS atmosphere is good | 26 | 74 | | | 0.000 | 0.462, 0.018 |
| CS is well accepted | 50 | 50 | | | 0.013 | 0.555, 0.000 |
| *Perception* | Yes | No | | | | |
| Performed by doctor in any specialty | 19 | 81 | | | - | - |
| CS in HK is safe | 50 | 50 | | | 0.115 | - |
| Botox injection is CS | 61 | 39 | | | 0.243 | - |
| Pleasure resulted | 48 | 52 | | | 0.000 | - |
| CS in future | 30 | 70 | | | 0.000 | - |
| Permanency | 32 | 68 | | | 0.105 | - |
| Discrimination after CS | 22 | 61 | | | 0.000 | 0.495, 0.023 |
| CSC | Beauty center | Medical beauty center | Aesthetic surgery center | | 0.001 | 0.284, 0.003 |
| | 12 | 35 | 53 | | | |
| Reasons | Increase social competitively | Increase self confidence | Flaw improvement | | 0.058 | - |
| | 3 | 41 | 52 | | | |

[a] Totals may be <100 because of missing values.

# RESULTS

Results for the prevalence of personal, social and perception variables are shown. Age, income, education, family, media, atmosphere, acceptance, CSC, happiness, and objection were positively associated with CS, while age, income, education, family, media, atmosphere, acceptance, centers, and objection were the only variables positively associated with CS addiction (Table 1).

# DISCUSSION

As the result of personal variables, we are able to explain the popularity of surgery as being caused by the fact that more and more people who are dissatisfied with their appearance can afford to change their physical appearance (Watts, 2004). The marital status variable was not associated with CS in our study, possibly due to the fact that the social status of females has changed. Married or divorced women may please their husbands or increase their "marketability" by having CS. This may affect the thinking and the health of the next generation.

The results of social variables, phi coefficient and approx. sig. of the family variables were 0.733 and 0.001, which is the highest compared to other variables. As the value of 0.733 is approaching 1, this means there is a very close relationship between family factors and addiction. It was noted that mothers brought their daughters to the clinic and it was probably the mothers who asked them to undergo CS, even though the girls did not really know what they were doing (Lok, 2007) reflecting that the family element must be the core consideration in the health education and promotion of CS.

The rate of CS media attraction, at 37%, was larger than "family" at 20%, but the Phi coefficient and approx. sig. of media were 0.478 and 0.004, not as high as for family (0.733 and p=0.001). Although the media effect on use of CS is high, it does not have a strong correlation with CS addiction. The results from the present study contrast with the previous report of a 20.6% effect by the family and a 13.3% media effect. It may be caused by changes in social norms. A variety of CS advertisements can be found in different media (The Standard, 2006) where are often accused of unrealistic expectations/portrayals of female beauty (Polonijo & Carpiano, 2008). Consistent with our results, other studies have also found a small positive association between CS makeover program viewing and desire to undergo CS procedure (Harrsion, 2003; Bandura, 1986). Media depictions have the ability to influence human behavior without our awareness, and to influence individuals' decisions (Alba, 2000).

Social variables, atmosphere (0.462, p=0.018) and acceptance (0.555, p=0.000) show a positive but not too strong correlation with CS addiction. Interestingly, 74% think the social norm ("atmosphere" variable) of CS is not good, but 50% think CS is well accepted. It may reflect that Hong Kong females think that CS, although not good, is common. Many women around us have undergone CS in secret, as Hong Kong people are still quite conventional. 137 complaints were received by the Television and Entertainment Licensing Authority after the launch of the CS program that supported our result (Singtao, 2007). It is dangerous that the public may not have understood CS well before the operation.

**Table 2. Suicide due to appearance since 2007 in Hong Kong**

| Date | Case |
|------|------|
| 2010/03/03 | 23 years old, Hong Kong University student who has acnes and emotional suffered. |
| 2009/12/16 | 28 years old teenage who was marred by a dentist in 2001. Got a serious depression and tried suicide twice. Finally he sued the dentist for $1.7 millions. |
| 2008/09/02 | A twelve year old, form 2 girl died because her appearance was against by school. |
| 2007/06/04 | 14 years old girl who has eczema and was bullied by classmates to cause suicide. |

Only a minority answered correctly that CS in Hong Kong can be performed by doctor in any specialty (HKACCS, 2008). This misleads the public into feeling completely safe in undergoing CS and neglecting the health risks before their operation. Health education and promotion should be enforced in these aspects. We also found that 50% agreed that CS in Hong Kong is safe, implying that there is still room for improvement to the image of the CS industry. Also, 61% think Botox or hyaluronic acid injection constitutes CS. Although such injections are non-surgical CS, 39% may disapprove of the "aftermath". Apart from increasing the public's knowledge of CS through health education and promotion, it is suggested that the industry cooperate with the media to raise industrial transparency with the goad of smooth development of commercial CS (Fraser, 2003). Additionally, there is still a large portion, nearly 50%, who will not choose an aesthetic surgery center. In fact, CS specialists seldom stay in beauty centers and medical beauty centers. Sometimes, CS is practiced by somebody who is trained only in that area and is not even a medical practitioner. It may also increase the chance of accidents. Crisis management must be undertaken by the industry due to the unclear regulations and legislation. Besides, 32% think CS is permanent. In fact, this is not necessarily the case. The biological composition of the body cannot be fully controlled or manipulated because it is embedded in physical limitations that influence one's appearance (Ricciardelli & Clow, 2009).

Nearly 50% think CS can give you pleasure and affects your normal daily activities, which shows the potential to become addicted. From our findings, 27% have tried CS and 30% will consider trying it in the near future. It is observed from the three-way cross-tabulation that 19% have had CS and been satisfied with the results, and will try it again in the near future. The Phi coefficient is 0.558 and approx. sig. is 0.000, showing a strong correlation among the three predictors with significance. People may suffer Body Dysmorphic Disorder, which may lead to further aesthetic surgery (Reich, 1991).

52% think CS is caused by flaw improvement; 41% would like to increase their self-confidence, and 3% would like to increase their social competitiveness. That means most are persuaded by the perfectionist (Chrisler, 2007), western ideals of beauty (Watts, 2004), and more than 40% lack self-confidence. Studies suggest that low self-esteem and feeling judged on one's physical appearance may lead individuals to consider CS (Davis, 2002). Patients seek CS when a long holiday has been reported, so as to gain self-confidence and more easily improve competitiveness and occupation (Watts, 2004). No pain, no gain. Physical and psychological health risks must be involved. Laziness (Lerner, 1969) resulting from CS may reduce the healthy eating and exercise to cause poor physical health. Others like pain, bruising, blood loss or infections are common, occurring in up to one in four breast augmentation patients (Gabriel et al., 1997). Common postoperative psychological consequences include anxiety, disappointment, and depression (Borah et al., 1999). For the worst, the mortality rate for CS is approximately 1 in 13,000, comparable to that for general surgical procedures (Yoho et al., 2005). But deaths from liposuction, 20 per 100,000, are comparable to motor vehicle accidents at 16.4 per 100,000 (Grazer & de Jong, 2000). There may also be a risk of suicide caused by failed CS. The body is conceptualized as a "project" (Goffman, 1968) that is modified as a fundamental part of self-identity (Shilling, 2003) to increase confidence and ideal beauty. Furthermore, according to Festinger's (1954) social comparison theory, people compare themselves to others (Blum, 2005) for self-improvement and self-enhancement (Wood, 1989), both of which have direct relevance for issues of body image and appearance. But the beauty trend will change with time. Non-stop surgeries will take place, easily triggering addiction.

On the other hand, we found a medium strong correlation with discrimination or objection and CS addiction. This can be explained by the fact that agreement or appreciation would be gained from others after surgery. However, negative results may stimulate junkies.

Although CS does bring negative health risks to public, it can also positively impact or help to prevent tragedies. There has been at least one suicide owing to bad appearance in Hong Kong since 2007 (Table 2) (The Sun, 2010). It has been reported that 15% of depressed teenagers will commit suicide if they suffer from a problematic appearance for a long time (The Sun, 2010). CS has emerged as an increasingly by popular option for women who want to look better and subsequently boost their emotional well-being (Grossbart & Sarwer, 2003).

CS is now being transformed to survive and thrive as an essential part of 21st century health care. We suggest that the cosmetic, psychological, and psychiatric elements be enhanced in the curriculum in order for the healthcare professions to be better equipped for plastic surgery. CS should also provide comprehensive healthcare services. Final year medical students have a designated attachment to the Division of Plastic, Reconstructive and Aesthetic Surgery (Burd et al., 2004). Specialists' and nurses' care are equally important to the public too. We advise offering such designated courses to nursing students in the coming future.

In fact, the importance of appearance is somehow nibbling away at society and public health. A team of registered nurses can be formed and trained to specialize in appearance and cosmetic aspects which seem to be essential tools for preventing the above tragedies. Cosmetic, counseling, psychiatric and psychological skills could be enhanced in such a specialized training course for nurses to change patients' perceptions of themselves and facilitate improvement in their psychological functioning (Pruzinsky, 1993) thorough school seminar. The most serious and problematic student cases can be helped by CS with parental and medical agreement. Suicide is not the only way to solve a problem. In order to prevent CS abuse and addiction, screening must be done, and that can also be practiced by nurses. Nurses can play an important role as a bridge between the primary care team and different sectors (Figure 1). We suggest that a professional certificate or diploma course, curriculum with other related industries, continuous education credits in cosmetic aspects could be further considered to provide better service, reduce health risks and consolidate the whole CS system.

The CS, health and beauty care industries are closely related. Post-care like massage and firming treatments after liposuction can be treated by the beauty industry to share the resources and the overlapping areas.

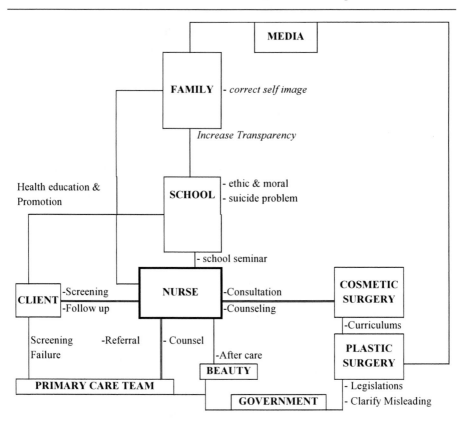

Figure 1. Collaboration in cosmetic industry.

A disclaimer is usually signed by the patient before CS in a CSC. Insurance may not be claimed for CS when something goes wrong, because much CS is not done by specialists in plastic surgery. Insurance bought from a general practitioner may not cover CS likes insurance bought by specialists in plastic surgery from the Medical Protection Society Limited.

Four foreseeable trends of CS in Hong Kong are found. First, its acceptance and development must be increased in the coming years (HKACCS, 2008). Second, the age of CS patients will be younger (China News, 2008). Third, males will be the target of the CS industry. One out of four of patients is a male (Lok, 2007). Lower confidence in men significantly predicted willingness to undergo CS (Ricciardelli & Clow,

2009). Fourth, repair of CS will be the mainstream of the industry if no further improvements are made.

Our study has some limitations. Because of its cross sectional design, we cannot draw conclusions about causal relations between the variables examined. Although the response rate was over 60%, the sample size was still not large enough to prevent a sampling error, which lowers the validity. Because of the sensitivity and privacy of Hong Kong women, it was hard to find respondents. Another limitation is that non-probability snowball sampling was adopted, which was not due to random chance and which can result in significant bias. We were also unable to widen the older age group, because questionnaires were distributed by electronic means, which may have restricted the sample age groups: older people may not use computers in their everyday lives. It is suggested that a different data collection method be used next time. The small sampling size makes statistical work difficult. We are unable to generalize our results. Large sample recruitment could be tried with stakeholders so as to study Hong Kong CS in greater depth, and prediction of CS risk factors can be done by logistic regression in the future. Finally, we were unable to specify terms in detail to conduct a more accurate studies.

## CONCLUSION

In conclusion, we found a concrete picture of CS for Hong Kong females. Different correlates of CS and addiction were explored. These findings may suggest that CS affects daily life and health in ways that are crucial to offer insights for health education and promotion on CS and addiction. We also found that training and support of specialties, nurses, beauticians and the primary health care team should be available to meet the demand and supply in Hong Kong. A multi-sectional curriculum should be prepared to support all the professionals who will cooperate together. Nurses can play an important role in bridging different sectors and screening in the CS aspect. Better health education and promotion can then be worked out so that beauty junkies can be prevented. And it is hoped that other researchers will study this area more in order to benefit the health of Hong Kong society.

# REFERENCES

Alba, J.W. (2000). Dimensions of consumer expertise. *Advances in Consumer Research, 27,*1-9.

Bandura, A. (1986). *Social foundations of thought and action: A social cognitive theory.* Englewood Cliffs (NJ): Prentice-Hall.

Blum, V. (2005). Becoming the Other Woman. The Psychic Drama of Cosmetic Surgery. *Frontiers,* 26.

Borah, G., Rankin, M., & Wey, P. (1999). Psychological complications in 281 surgery practices. *Plastic & Reconstructive Surgery, 104,*1241-1246.

Burd, A., Chiu, T., & McNaught, C. (2004). Plastic surgery in the undergraduate curriculum: the importance of considering students' perceptions. *Br J Plast Surg, 57,*773-779.

China News. (2008). Nearly 400 females for breast augmentation in Hong Kong. Retrieved August 12, 2009, from http://www.chinanews.com

Chrisler, J.C. (2007) Presidential address: fear of losing control: power, perfectionism, and the psychology of women. Psychology of *Women Quarterl, 32,*1-12.

Consumer Council. (2007). Council exposes myths in beauty treatment of double eyelids - CHOICE # 373. Retrieved August 13, 2009, from http://www.consumer.org.hk/website/ws_en/news/press_releases/p373 02.html

Consumer Council. (2008). Council debunks myths of self-claimed "non-surgical cosmetic treatments" - CHOICE # 375. Retrieved August 13, 2009, from http://www.consumer.org.hk/website/ws_en/news/press_ releases/p37502.html

Davis, K. (2002). 'A dubious equality': Men, women and cosmetic surgery. *Body and Society, 8,*49-65.

Festinger, L. (1954). A theory of social comparison process. *Human Relations, 7*,117-140.

Fraser, S. (2003). The Agent Within: Agency Repertories in Medical Discourse on Cosmetic Surgery. *Australian Feminist Studies, 18.*

Gabriel, S.E., Woods, J.E., O'Fallon, W.M., Beard, C.M., Kurland, L.T., & Melton, L.J.III. (1997). Complications leading to surgery after breast implantation. *New England Journal of Medicine, 336*,677-682.

Goffman, E. (1968). *The Presentation of Self in Everyday Life.* New York: Penguin.

Goodman, A. (2006). Addiction: definition and implications. *Addiction, 85*,1403-1408.

Grazer, F.M., & de Jong, R.H. (2000). Fatal outcomes from liposuction: Census survey of cosmetic surgeons. *Plastic & Reconstructive Surgery, 105*,436-446.

Grossbart, T.A., & Sarwer, D.B. (2003). Psychosocial issues and their relevance to the cosmetic surgery patient. *Seminars in Cutaneous Medicine and Surgery, 22*,136-147.

Harrsion, K. (2003). Television viewers' ideal body proportions: The case of the curvaceously thin woman. *Sex Roles, 48*,255-264.

HKACCS. (2007). Dr. To, the Secretary and Spokesman of HK Chapter of ACCS @ Cosmoprof Asia 2007 Seminar. Retrieved August 21, 2009, from http://www.accs.hk/files/Cosmoprof.pdf

HKACCS. (2008). The Specialization of Cosmetic Medicine. Retrieved August 20, 2009, from http://www.accs.hk/Media.html

Hong Kong Society of Plastic, Reconstructive and Aesthetic Surgeons. (2008). Plastic surgical specialty. Retrieved August 13, 2009, from http://www.plasticsurgery.org.hk/news_room.php

Hong Kong Trade Development Council. (2001). Beauty Business Looks Good. Retrieved November 20, 2008, from http://info.hktdc.com/imn/01092704/cosmetics03.htm?w_sid=194&w_pid=703&w_nid=&w_cid=&w_idt=1900-01-01&w_oid=207&w_jid=

Karnani, A. (2007). *Doing Well by Doing Good Case Study: 'Fair & Lovely' Whitening Cream.* University of Michigan.

Kumar, A., Godwin, J.W., & Gates, P.B. (2007). Molecular basis for the nerve dependence of limb regeneration in an adult vertebrate. *Science*, *318*,772-777.

Kwoh, L. (2006). The Standard: Quick fix turns into lifelong nightmare. Retrieved March 19, 2010, from http://www.thestandard.com.hk/news_detail.asp?we_cat=4&art_id=16579&sid=7508711&con_type=1&d_str=20060414

Lerner, R.M. (1969). Some female stereo-types of male body build-behavior relations. *Perceptual and Motor Skills*, *28*,363-366.

Lok, C. (2007). Culture and Leisure. In search of beauty. Retrieved August 17, 2009, from http://www.com.cuhk.edu.hk/varsity/0703/culture2a.htm

Markey, C., & Markey, P. (2009). Correlates of Young Women's Interest in Obtaining Cosmetic Surgery. *Sex Roles*, *61*,158-166.

Polonijo, A.N., & Carpiano, R.M. (2008). Representations of Cosmetic Surgery and Emotional Health in Women's Magazines in Canada. *Women's Health Issue*, *18*,463-470.

Pruzinsky, T. (1993). Psychological Factors in Cosmetic Plastic Surgery: Recent Developments in Patient Care. *American Society of Plastic Surgical Nursing*, *13*,64.

Reich, J. (1991). The Aesthetic Surgical Experience. In J.W.Smith & S.J.Ashton (eds.), Plastic Surgery. Boston.

Ricciardelli, R., & Clow, K. (2009). Men, Appearance, & Cosmetic Surgery: The Role of Self-Esteem And Comfort with The Body. *Canadian Journal of Sociology*, *34*.

Shilling, C. (2003). *The Body and Social Theory* (2nd ed.). London: Sage.

Singtao. (2007). 137 complaints received by Television and Entertainment Licensing Authority after launching the cosmetic surgery program which was sponsored by "Be A Lady" beauty company. Retrieved March 24, 2010, from http://www.singtao.com

The Sun. (2010). Ten-year-old girl is afraid of bullying and seeks cosmetic surgery. Retrieved March 15, 2010, from http://www.the-sun.on.cc/cnt/news/20100315/00410_001.html

Watts, J. (2004). China's cosmetic surgery craze. *The Lancet*, 958.

Wood, J. (1989). Theory and research concerning social comparisons of personal attributes. *Psychological Bulletin, 106,*231-248.

YWCA. (2004). Cosmetic Surgery and Slimming from Hong Kong Women. Retrieved August 13, 2009, from http://www.ywca.org.hk/research/200401a/news20040711.doc

Yoho, R.A., Romaine, J.J., & O'Neil, D. (2005). Review of the liposuction, abdominoplasty, and face-lift mortality and morbidity risk literature. *Dermatology Surgery, 31,*733-743.

*Chapter 2*

# EYELASH BEAUTY AND HEALTH

## *Zenobia C. Y. Chan and Queeni T. Y. Ip*
The Hong Kong Polytechnic University, China

## ABSTRACT

Eyelash beauty, including perming, extensions, dyeing, and tattoos, is popular around the world, where different races seek different treatments in order to achieve "electric" eyes according to the beauty definition of Western culture. Asian women generally favor eyelash perms and extensions. Eyelash beauty treatments are assumed to improve ethnic "deficiencies" and bring psychological benefits in terms of femininity, normalcy and self management. Frequent treatments and chemical products place stress on the eye and are closely related to a person's health in general. Issues pertaining to the ethnic differences in eyelashes, the reasoning behind seeking out the procedure, physical health risks and women's positive feelings toward eyelash beauty are illustrated. The negative impact on women's beauty is also implicated. There is a lack of literature about eyelash beauty and women's health. This article aims to enable better understanding of Asian beauty and some of the implications for women's health.

# INTRODUCTION

Eyelashes are the hairs that grow at the edges of the eyelid to protect the eye from debris; they are sensitive to being touched, thus providing a warning that an object is near the eye. They start beneath the skin near the muscles of the eyelids, which are responsible for opening and closing the lids. Their actions are synergistically coordinated by signals from the nervous system in the normal, healthy person (International Society of Hair Restoration Surgery, 2007).

Long and voluminous eyelashes are seen as a sign of femininity and beauty in many cultures. Hadza women are known to trim their own eyelashes (Hadza, 2003). Kohl was worn as far back as the Bronze Ages to protect and enhance lashes. In ancient Egypt, it was used by the wealthy and royalty to protect their eyes from sand, dust and bugs. Modern women seek to enhance their eyelashes artificially by using mascara and false lashes. The beginning of the popularity of convincing-looking false eyelashes was in the 1960s. Eyelash beauty mainly refers to perms, extensions, dyeing and tattooing (Hornblass, 1988) that give volume to the lashes; such treatments have become popular in salons (Xinhuanet, 2006).

Apart from the above salon treatment, home care eyelash products are very common. The rapid development of eyelash conditioners, which increase the health and length of lashes, has been seen in the past decade. Many seed extracts, minerals, and other chemicals are used in eyelash conditioners to achieve the desired results. Other popular eyelash products like mascara also contain an abundance of chemicals. It is indicated that the glue used for false eyelashes might cause irritation and infection (Consumer Council, 2007). However, people seldom think about the possibility of such eyelash products harming their health. In addition, it is worth seeking out the reasons behind women's pursuit of eyelash beauty so as to gain a better understanding for the planning of women's health promotion and education.

Literature related to eyelashes mostly covers hypertrichosis and pigmentation (Johnstone, 1997; Wand, 1997), reflection and eyelash detection (Kang & Park, 2007; Kong & Zhang, 2001; 2003), oncology

(Annals of Oncology, 2005), ophthalmology (Noda et al., 1989), immunodeficiency (Kaplan et al., 1991), latanoprost treatment (Mansberger & Cioffi, 2000), hair transplantation in plastic surgery, and related disorders (Choi & Kim, 2004; Marritt, 1980; Rubin & Warner, 1997; Schmidt, 1997; Tyers & Collin, 2001).

Eyelash cosmetics are seldom mentioned (Draelos, 1995). Interesting topics like chemical cosmetics, the health risks behind eyelash cosmetics, the ethnic differences in eyelashes, the reasons for eyelash beauty, the smart buys in eyelash products, etc. are rarely found. However, these topics all closely relate to human health, especially that of women. These mascaras can run under the effect of tears, but are easily removed with some soap and water. Polymers in a water-dispersed form (latexes) can bring some level of water resistance to the group of normally non-water resistant mascaras. The waxy components of waterproof mascara, which can weaken the eyelash, are proportionally greater than in the non-waterproof versions. Although non-waterproof mascara does not function as well as waterproof mascara, it is relatively more healthy for the eyelash. It is important to know what chemicals are contained in cosmetics and their impact on eyelash health.

In fact, it has been shown that eyelash products like glues are examined only if they bear adequate labeling information for proper use. Nearly half of the samples bore no user instructions in Chinese or English on their labels. Further, as some glues may be inflammable or emit flammable gases, consumers should not smoke or get too close to a source of fire when applying the glue. However, only a few samples carried such a caution on flammability. Inadequate labeling information increases the risk of the glue accidentally getting into the eyes or catching fire, thus manufacturers and suppliers are urged to review the labeling information on their products. Ophthalmologists have stressed the importance of proper application to prevent the glue getting into the eyes. Instead of reusing artificial eyelashes, it is more advisable to use a new pair to avoid infection. People with eye infections should avoid wearing contact lens and makeup altogether (Consumer Council, 2008).

There is evidence that in a Consumer Council test on 40 mascara samples, two mascaras were detected with a total bacterial count of 78,000 cfu/g, which is more than 150 times the permitted limit (standard plate count) of 500 cfu/g or per ml based on the mainland's Hygiene Standard for Cosmetics. The use of unhygienic mascara may greatly increase the risk of developing eye infection or inflammation. Excessive levels of microbial content in cosmetics may be due to a host of reasons. In both cases, the two mascara samples were not labeled with any information in relation to their manufacturing and/or expiry dates. Consumers have therefore no clue as to the hygiene condition of these products, or if the products are beyond expiration for use.

The Hong Kong Medical Association has advised people to stop using make-up when they feel irritation in the eyes, and to use appropriate tools to remove mascara thoroughly. Highlighted in the report were three medical cases attended by doctors. A patient was found with a few eyelashes hidden under her lower eyelid. The eyelashes had apparently fallen off during the make-up removal process and remained in the eyes, causing irritation. Another patient felt unwell in her eyes for nearly half a year; on examination, it was found that she had been taking a make-up training course, and that she might have shared contaminated cosmetics with other classmates, resulting in irritation of the eyes. In the third case, the patient felt itchiness after applying eye make-up, and her eyes became red and swollen; the irritation was later found to be caused by certain ingredients in the eye cosmetics (Consumer Council, 2007).

Much has been written about cosmetics and eyelash health. Waterproof mascara and eye makeup are some of the most common causes of eyelash loss. These products are notoriously difficult to remove and cling to the lashes like glue. Harshly rubbing and pulling on lashes to remove mascara is a sure-fire way to cause the eyelashes to fall out in clumps. A Staphylococcus aureus infection causes eyelashes not only to fall out, but also to grow back in different directions. Parasitic mite infections and syphilis are other common eye infections that cause lashes to fall out. On the other hand, hormonal changes in the amount of thyroid hormones cause metabolic disturbances that can change hair growth and structure. The eyelash cell cycle is affected, causing lashes to become thin, break, and shorten. The end result is that eyelashes look like they are falling out in patches and clumps. Certainly another common cause of eyelash loss can be from drugs, such as chemotherapy for cancer patients (Minogue, 2009).

Eye cosmetics are without doubt an important part of facial make-up. Care should always be exercised to avoid injury (Consumer Council, 2007). The trend to seek eyelash beauty is long and complex. The majority of women, especially Asians, are looking to enhance their feminine characteristics. It is obvious that the hair of Asians is not as long, curly or dark compared to that of other races (NHI, 1997). Apart from protection by shielding the eye from injury like that caused by dust and grit, another principal function of the eyelashes for modern humans is ornamental. Like other facial features, they create an appearance that is unique to every individual. A person without eyelashes has an abnormal appearance because they are lacking one of the important anatomical landmarks of facial normality. Additionally, the ornamental value of eyelashes is subject to fashion trends that decree what "look" is preferred in any given era and culture (International Society of Hair Restoration Surgery, 2007). Such trends are cultivated by the advent of movies and television in our daily life. We are told to strive for "contemporary" femininity, control and self management through female beauty. Therefore, pursuing eyelash beauty has become a hot trend.

Asian women are motivated to improve on that issue so that they can restore femininity, normalcy, and a complete sense of self. The development of better eyelash treatment techniques and products is therefore increasing. However, the health knowledge behind and precautions regarding these techniques and products are neglected. The purpose of the article was to analyze different eyelash beauty for different types of women, to explore the physical and psychological reasons why Asian women are active in their pursuit of eyelash beauty, and to demonstrate appropriate care and precautions in eyelash care, especially for Asian women, so that oriental beauty and health can be upgraded and promoted.

## Ethnic Hair Differences

Eyelashes are one of the hair fibers known as specialized hairs. Their functions and structures are more or less the same as hair. Each individual is unique and hair production rate, size, and shape differs for everyone, but in general there are some differences in the nature of hair fiber for people of different ethnic backgrounds. They are mainly divided into Asian, Caucasian and African American. There will of course be small regional differences, but in general there are defined similarities among each of these ethnic groups. Hair type simply refers to color, texture and shape, and density. For color, dark hair is found in Africans and those of African descent (Belgravia Center, 2009); blonde, black, brown and red can be found in Caucasians (Belgravia Center, 2009); and Asians have black hair (NHI, 1997). For the texture and shape, the shape of the follicle is what determines the hair's shape. Asian hair is on average the thickest and most coarse hair compared to Caucasian and African hair. It is almost always straight and circular in cross section. Caucasian hair can be quite varied in its presentation, with straight, wavy or curly hair. The fiber can be circular or oval in cross section and is on average thinner than Asian hair. Finally, African hair is frequently tightly coiled, or spiral hair (Belgravia Center, 2009; Keratin, 2010; Khumalo et al., 2000). In cross section it is elliptical or almost flat and ribbon-like in some cases. This means that there is more strength and rigidity to the fiber across the area of greatest cross section, but the hair is much more pliable across the narrow section. This results in the curls of hair all naturally flexing and coiling along the ribbon, while there is little or no coiling from side to side (Keratin, 2010). Differences in hair density have been described according to ethnic background, as well. Asians are known to have fewer hairs than Caucasians (Keratin, 2010; Lee et al., 2002). The density of hair follicles in Africans is also somewhat lower than for Caucasians on average (Keratin, 2010; Loussouarn, 2001; Sperling, 1999). The density of Asian hair may be just 90,000 scalp follicles and rarely gets above 120,000 scalp follicles, while the hair density of Caucasians can range from 100,000 to 150,000 scalp hair follicles.

## Asian Eyelash Beauty

Asians, especially women, are active in seeking eyelash beauty since the nature of their eyelashes is relatively darker, shorter, thicker, coarser and less dense, which are not the standards of modern western eyelash beauty. Montague (1968) showed that long curved eyelashes do indeed enhance a woman's beauty. However, the worst eyelash problem for Asians is that the emergent angle of Asian hair is less acute. Asian hair emerges slightly more perpendicular to the skin and thus appears to stand away from the scalp. Interestingly, hair in Asian newborns often stands straight up. When Asian hair is long, the heavy weight of the thick shafts tends to bend it down, so it will not be curly enough, but bent hair fortunately always looks fuller than straight and flat hair. Therefore, Asians tend to seek eyelash perms and extensions, while Caucasians prefer eyelash dyeing and tattoos owing to the high skin to hair color contrast (NHI, 1997).

## Eyelash Perms and Extensions

Apart from using eye cosmetic aids, false lashes, eyelash curlers, eyelash curlkeepers, mascara and eyelash serum, etc. to give an impression of "Caucasian eyes", eyelash beauty for Asians is mainly achieved by perms and extensions, which can create a larger, more round eye shape with longer and more dense eyelashes. Eyelash dyeing and tattooing are also available in beauty salons.

The principles and concepts of hair and eyelash perms are similar. 30 minutes should be enough for an eyelash perm, which is not as long as that for hair perms, and the curl can then last four to eight weeks. This is relatively more convenient and time-saving when compared with the eyelash curler. It is also good for women who need eye makeup every day, as they usually apply eye makeup with "capricious" hands, even doing so in public transport in order to save time. Application tools with sharp edges may also easily hurt the eyes and cornea (Consumer Council, 2008).

Eyelashes can be weakened and easily broken if not curled properly every day.

Different styles of eyelash waving can be requested, as with hair perm. Different degrees of eyelash perm can give different styles of eyelash. Such different shapes show different characteristics and match with different facial features so that different personal images can be formed. Eyelash design experts will design different styles. They can mainly be divided into three different levels: the energetic tighter curl, the lovely all around curl and the natural longer lash or looser curl, which is the type that men prefer. Although eyelash perms are not common for Asian men, they can be helpful for abnormal or ingrown eyelashes. It has been observed that different clients give equal preference to these different curls in the beauty salon. In recent years, the techniques for eyelash perm have been developed and improved, so that more natural and longer lashes result. This is because different rods are used and, since eyelash perms control the direction of the lashes, they can sometimes give the impression of greater length. In addition, random directional growth in the lashes can be corrected by an eyelash perm as well. If eyelash length appears to be uneven because the way that the eyelashes curl is not uniform, an eyelash perm can help. However, extending the eyelashes is the best way to create an even and uniform length in the lash hairs.

Eyelash extensions are the most effective way of adding actual length to short lashes. Although the eyelash perm gives the impression of greater length, the impression is still not markedly different if the eyelashes are very short. The added volume from eyelash extensions can also sometimes hide the random directional growth in the lashes. Besides, it will immediately add volume to thin lashes. Applying extensions is appropriate as long as the lashes are strong enough to support the weight of the extensions and adhesive. Adding extensions darker than your natural shade of hair will also make the lashes appear darker, and will add fullness to the eyelash. Perming or dyeing the lashes a darker color can also give the illusion of volume, although this is usually not as dramatic as with eyelash extension. This is the best option if you are generally happy with the look of your lashes, other than their color, and want to reduce the need for mascara (SHIZUKA New York Day Spa, 2010).

## Eyelash Transplantation

Eyelash transplant surgeries may help to reconstruct or thicken lashes. As the availability and success of eyelash transplantation becomes better known, more people, more often women than men, are considering the surgical approach to gain permanent enhancement of eyelash length and density. Eyelash transplantation for esthetic facial enhancement is a relatively recent development. It is believed that the number of cases will increase with the social acceptance of cosmetic surgery in Asia.

## DISCUSSION

Physical ethnic "deficiencies" cause Asian women to seek eyelash beauty in order to achieve the pervasive Western female beauty cultural norms. The Miss Chinatown USA beauty pageant has actually been found to use white standards to judge Chinese-American women, prompting one community member to state her belief that the contest showed that the more you look like a White, the prettier you are. Also, these Asian Americans tended to internalize the "white standards" of beauty promoted by the mass media. "Caucasian" eyes represented a standard of beauty for Chinese-American contestants, who curled their eyelashes (Scranton, 2001). From a feminist or cultural perspective, women's beauty is equated with competence, self-control, intelligence, and feminine voluptuousness (in particular, large breasts), with wide-eyed, giggly vapidity. Like the processes through which "docile" and "subjected" femininity is shaped by the "tyranny of slenderness", an appearance-directed normative imperative is revealed in the constitution of the feminine self. As a metaphor for the correct management of desire throughout the dominant Western religious and philosophical traditions, the capacity for self-management is decisively coded as male (Bordo, 1993).

Popular culture does continue to rearrange and self-transform. We are constantly told that we can "choose" our own bodies. At the other extreme, it is being just as unequivocally declared that "Bodies are not born. They are in fact made by culture." People pursue happiness on the terms of the culture in which they live. But, they also want to feel that they are self-determining agents, and some also want to be reassured that their choices are "politically correct".

We believe that such beautification is continually mystified in the commercial constructions of body alteration as self-determination and creative self-fashioning (Bordo, 1993). We have learned that such cultures, control, and self management are all cultivated by the advent of movies and television in our daily life. Bordo points out that the rules for femininity have come to be culturally transmitted more and more through standardized visual images. Contemporary advertisements reveal continual and astute manipulation of problems that psychology and the popular media have targeted as characteristic dilemmas of the "contemporary woman" beset by conflicting role demands and pressures on her time. For example, in the ad slogan for mascara: "Perfect Pen Eyeliner Puts You in Control. And isn't that nice for a change?", the word "control" was used. "Mastery" also figures frequently in ads for cosmetics and hair products. "Master your curls with new Adaptable Perm." We are told to control, master or manage our life through the normalizing culture of female beauty. Ultimately, the body is seen as demonstrating correct/ incorrect attitudes toward the demands of normalization itself. Female bodies become docile bodies whose forces and energies are habituated to external regulation, subjection, transformation, and "improvement". The relatively short and less dense lashes of Chinese women can be "improved" by different kinds of eyelash modifications, which implies that we continue to memorize in our bodies the feeling and conviction of insufficiency and never being good enough. At the farthest extremes, the practices of femininity may lead us to an utterly negative health impact like cosmetic addiction in women. It was worrying that the cosmetic addition caused by the constant reminder of short and less dense hair drew attention to the necessity of perpetual self-monitoring. Bordo (1993) also suggested that body regimes weaken women's position of power in society, although she argues that practices designed to control and discipline women's behaviors, such as dietary regimes and intensive body building, produce an obedient and submissive feminine body, even if some women experience these techniques as empowering.

Eyelash beauty treatment results in a "wide-awake" look, but the physical health risks and precautions should be addressed. As mentioned above, the waxy components cause the water-resistant effect of waterproof mascara. Stronger "detergent" is needed to remove the eye makeup. Such chemical and physical rubbing must compromise the eyelash health. Also, it has been observed that clients do not clean their lashes well, so that mascara residue is left. This may be because of an "effective" waterproof product or because a softer remover was used. It is not recommended to use facial makeup remover instead of that for the eyes. False lashes are very popular today. However, women should also be aware of the glue used, since irritation, inflammation and flammable problems of eye cosmetics can be caused by this component. Heavy "camouflage" increases the load on the eyelid and causes eye aging problems. Ophthalmologists advise that some people may be allergic to waterproof mascaras and should not use waterproof, glitter, lengthening and volumizing (thickening) mascara daily, as small particles may get into their eyes easily and increase the risk of eye infections, especially for those wearing contact lenses. They should shorten the time of wearing make-up, and use appropriate makeup remover and tools (i.e. cotton pads and rods) to remove waterproof cosmetics, as makeup residues may get into their eyes and cause irritation or even infections. Consumers should check the product label before buying and using, and dispose of eye cosmetics opened for a month, ceasing to use them if they dry out, deteriorate, or change color. They should not try to dilute dried mascaras with water, toner or other substances. The Consumer Council urges cosmetics manufacturers to include in the labeling comprehensive information on use-by dates, as well as ingredients, to facilitate consumers' choice. Other reasons for excessive microbial content in cosmetics are poor hygiene during the production process, damage to packaging, and insufficient or failure of preservatives in the products (Consumer Council, 2007; 2008).

The composition of eyelash products and some of the issues surrounding eyelash perms should also be brought to consumers' attention. Adverse reactions to perms are fairly rare but they do happen. The most common problem is lash damage. Perming involves some considerable rearrangement of biochemical bonds in the lash. If the process is performed inappropriately, it can permanently weaken the lash. In its mildest form, the damage presents as dull, coarse and lifeless. If the damage is very severe there may be significant eyelash breakage and loss. A diffuse thinning may occur and may not be uniform all over. There may be more damage in some areas than in others. If the lashes are damaged, eyelash serum is suggested. Perm kits should be used by professionals and technicians, but the public can easily access and buy them at drug stores and cosmetic stores. However, home users may not handle the products properly, ignoring the instructions and applying an inappropriate amount of the chemicals or applying them for too long. The concentration of the perm lotion may be different depending on the brand. And prices are different too. The age of the product is also an important determinant of how potent the chemicals are and how they affect the hair. If the chemicals are too weak or not left on the lashes for long enough, then inevitably the process will not take. If the neutralizer is not applied properly and not allowed to completely stop the hair biochemical bond breaking process of the thioglycolic acid, then the chemical bonds can gradually revert to their previous form. The chemicals involved are quite potent and they can damage the skin if left on for too long or if you have sensitive skin. Sometimes this can lead to an inflammatory skin reaction to the chemicals, whereby the skin can be itchy, red, and even painful in more severe cases. Sometimes this skin reaction can send the hair follicles into a telogen resting state. Hair follicles are fairly sensitive to skin inflammation, so if there is a lot of inflammation around they may shut down until the inflammation subsides. This can result in a thinning of the hair over the scalp. The hair follicles should recover and return to producing hair, but it may take them six months and sometimes longer to get back to normal. When in doubt, consumers should speak to their doctor. The most severe adverse response is a chemical burn. If the chemicals are left on the skin for too long there can be severe and irreversible damage. Chemical burns are pretty obvious at the time of the chemical exposure, as they should be quite painful. Users experiencing pain during the process should wash the chemicals off immediately.

The texture of lashes prior to application of the chemicals will affect the outcome of the process. Fine and limp lashes are usually more resistant to perming, and this type may need a stronger solution of chemicals or a longer exposure time to achieve the desired effect. Lashes that are wiry, brittle or damaged from another chemical process also resist waving. Because this kind of hair is already weaker than normal, there is a greater risk of hair breakage if the concentration of chemicals is made stronger. Special care is required to achieve good results and avoid severe damage.

It is recommended that eyelash perms be done by a professional in a beauty salon. It has also been observed that cheaper perm treatments are sometimes given by unlicensed trainees in some beauty salons. Further, the treatment price sometimes gives an indication of the quality of the perm lotion, which has a direct impact on your eyelash health and beauty. More information should be requested to assure health protection.

A popular myth claims that eyelash perms are less successful during menstruation and pregnancy. There is no actual evidence to prove that hair changes significantly during these periods. There may be an increase in oil production from the sebaceous glands that will subtly change the texture of hair, but that is all. Although the chemical processes involved in perms should still be fully effective, eyelash stylists should be concerned about using safe chemicals and products, as these have an impact on them too. It is not advised that pregnant women perm their hair or use too many chemical products. They can beautify their lashes using eyelash curlers or heat treatment. Proper care should always be taken to ensure eyelash health.

## CONCLUSION

Ethnic differences in hair features cause Asians actively to pursue eyelash perms and extensions that give the impression of "Caucasian" eyes, the beauty norm of the dominant Western culture. In this procedure, it is argued that female beauty is used to gain femininity, normalcy, self management and empowerment. In contrast, it is noted that there are many health risks inherent in eyelash beauty treatments, especially the cosmetic addiction caused by the constant reminder of short and less dense hair and drawing attention to the necessity of perpetual self-monitoring. The public should understand these clearly before seeking such treatments, and should be aware of the need to take some precautions. Eyelash cosmetics are seldom mentioned in the eyelash literature. This article aims to upgrade and promote oriental women's health and beauty by stimulating a discussion on the perception of eyelash beauty. There are still many areas to be explored. It is hoped that this article will stimulate further related study to promote a deeper understanding of women's health.

## REFERENCES

Annals of Oncology. (2005). Trichomegaly of the eyelashes following treatment with cetuximab. Retrieved Jan 12, 2010, from http://annonc.oxfordjournals.org/cgi/reprint/mdi300v1.pdf

Belgravia Center. (2009). Hair Types and Race Differences. Retrieved Jan 11, 2010, from http://www.belgraviacenter.com/blog/hair-types-and-race-differences/

Bordo, S. (1993). *Unbearable Weight, Feminism, Western Culture and the Body*. Berkeley: University of California Press.

Choi, Y.C., & Kim, J.C. (2004). Hair transplantation: Eyebrow, *eyelash*, mustache, and pubic area hair transplantation. New York.

Consumer Council. (2004). Press Releases: Hair dyes vary in safety levels as risk assessment study gets underway - CHOICE # 331. Retrieved

Jan 13, 2010, from http://www.consumer.org.hk/website/ws_en/news /press_releases/p33102.html

Consumer Council. (2007). Press Releases: Two mascaras found in excess of safety standard on microbial content - CHOICE # 370. Retrieved Jan 13, 2010, from http://www.consumer.org.hk/website/wsen/news/ press_releases/ p37001.html

Consumer Council. (2008). Press Releases: Test clears glues for cosmetic use of formaldehyde concern - CHOICE # 383. Retrieved Jan 13, 2010, from http://www.consumer.org.hk/website/ws_en/news/press_releases/p383 04.html

Draelos, Z.D. (1995). Cosmetics in dermatology. *Eyelash Cosmetics.* New York: Churchill Livingstone.

"Hadza". 2003. *Encyclopedia of sex and gender: men and women in the world's cultures, Volume 1.* New York: Springer.

Hornblass, A. (1988). Eyelids (Oculoplastic, Orbital and Reconstructive Surgery, Vol 1). Williams & Wilkins.

International Society of Hair Restoration Surgery. (2007). Eyelash Transplantation: Who, Why and How. Retrieved Jan 07, 2010, from http://www.ishrs.org/articles/eyelash-transplantation.htm

Johnstone, M.A. (1997). Hypertrichosis and increased pigmentation of eyelashes and adjacent hair in the region of the ipsilateral eyelids of patients treated with unilateral topical latanoprost. *American Journal of Ophthalmology, 124*(4),544-547.

Kang, B.J., & Park, K.R. (2007). A robust eyelash detection based on iris focus assessment. *Elsevier, 28*(13),1630-1639.

Kaplan, M.H., Sadick, N.S., & Talmor, M. (1991). Acquired trichomegaly of the eyelashes: a cutaneous marker of acquired immunodeficiency syndrome. *Journal of the American Academy of Dermatology, 25*(5),801-804.

Keratin. (2010). Ethnic differences in hair fiber and hair follicles. Retrieved Jan 12, 2010, from http://www.keratin.com/aa/aa002.shtml

Khumalo, N.P., Doe, P.T., Dawber, R.P., & Ferguson, D.J. (2000). What is normal black African hair? A light and scanning electron-microscopic study. *J Am Acad Dermatol, 43* (5.1),814-820.

Kong, W.K., & Zhang, D. (2001). Accurate Iris Segmentation Based on Novel Reflection and Eyelash Detection Model. Biometrics Technology Center, Department of Computing, The Hong Kong Polytechnic University.

Kong, W.K., & Zhang, D. (2003). Detecting eyelash and reflection for accurate iris segmentation. *International Journal of Pattern Recognition and Artificial Intelligence, 17*(6),1025-1034.

Lee, H.J., Ha, S.J., Lee, J.H., Kim, J.W., & Kim, H.O. (2002). Whiting DA. Hair counts from scalp biopsy specimens in Asians. *J Am Acad Dermatol, 46*(2),218-221.

Loussouarn, G. (2001). African hair growth parameters. *Br J Dermatol, 145*(2),294-297.

Mansberger, S.L., & Cioffi, G.A. (2000). Eyelash Formation Secondary to Latanoprost Treatment in a Patient With Alopecia. *Arch Ophthalmol, 118*(5),718-719.

Marritt, E. (1980). Transplantation of single hairs from the scalp as eyelashes. Review of the literature and a case report. *J Dermatol Surg Oncol,* 6(4),271-273.

Minogue, K. (2009). Why Are My Eyelashes Falling Out? Common Medical Causes and How You Can Stop Eyelash Fall Out. Retrieved Jan 07, 2010, from http://ezinearticles.com/?Why-Are-My-Eyelashes-Falling-Out?--Common-Medical-Causes-and-How-You-Can-Stop-Eyelash-Fall-Out&id=2837055

New Hair Institute, NHI. (1997). Racial Variations. Retrieved Jan 11, 2010, from http://www.newhair.com/treatment/fut-racial-variations.asp

Noda, S., Hayasaka, S., & Setogawa, T. (1989). Epiblepharon with inverted eyelashes in Japanese children. I. Incidence and symptoms. *Br J Ophthalmol, 73,*126-127.

Rubin, P.A.D., & Warner, M.A. (1997). Facial surgery: plastic and reconstructive: *Eyelash* and Eyebrow Disorders. Baltimore: Williams & Wilkins.

Scranton, P. (2001). Beauty and business: commerce, gender, and culture in modern America. Routledge: New York.

Schmidt, E.E. (1997). Lids and nasolacrimal system: clinical procedures. *Eyelash* Disorders and Procedures. Boston: Butterworth-Heinemann.

SHIZUKA New York Day Spa. (2010). Choosing between Eyelash Perms, Extensions and Eyelash Tinting. Retrieved Jan 13, 2010, from http://www.shizukany.com/fix-my-eyelashes.htm

Sperling, L.C. (1999). Hair density in African Americans. *Arch Dermatol, 135*(6),656-658.

Tan, M. (2002). *How to attract Asian Women.* New York.

Tyers, A.G.., & Collin, J.R.O. (2001). *Colour atlas of ophthalmic plastic surgery: Eyelash Abnormalities.* Oxford, Boston: Butterworth-Heinemann.

Wand, M. (1997). Latanoprost and Hyperpigmentation of Eyelashes. *Arch Ophthalmol, 115*(9),1206-1208.

Xinhuanet. (2006). Plug and sew eyelashes for women. Retrieved Jan 07, 2010, from http://news.xinhuanet.com/english/2006-10/25/content_5248767.htm

*Chapter 3*

# EYEBROW BEAUTY AND HEALTH

## *Zenobia C. Y. Chan and Queeni T. Y. Ip*
The Hong Kong Polytechnic University, China

## ABSTRACT

Eyebrow beauty treatments are commonly available in Hong Kong salons and elsewhere. Although there is literature addressing the eyebrows from an aesthetic point of view, these articles are seldom related to health. However, it is important to address the health risks of such treatments because of their popularity. In addition, eyebrow beauty, especially the eyebrow tattoo, is seen as a "self-injury", which internalizes women's psychological health risk. It is argued that female beauty is a self-normalization to feminine culture so as to achieve internal stability. In contrast, failure and such oppressive societal norms of beauty and femininity are hypothesized as a big bomb that ultimately weakens social mental health. This article describes eyebrow beauty and women's health. Its aim is to promote beauty and health for women by studying the eyebrow beauty, especially tattooing; finding out the reasons for the pursuit of eyebrow beauty; and exploring the associated health risks. Health educators and providers may find these helpful when designing prevention and intervention strategies for women's beauty.

# INTRODUCTION

The eyebrows provide physical protection to the eyes and play an important role in facial attractiveness (Cosio & Robins, 2000), sexual dimorphism (Bruce et al., 1993), nonverbal communication and emotional expression (Ekman, 1979). Different shapes of eyebrows give different images, and eyebrow thickness was found to play an important role in discriminating between male and female faces (Bruce et al., 1993). Relative thinness of the eyebrows might serve as part of a quick diagnostic of juveniles, females, and fine-featured males. Also, there is evidence to show the importance of the eyebrows as a mechanism of face recognition in humans. All the above reasons contribute to the popularity of eyebrow beauty. Bordo (1993) said that women's bodies are seen as "speaking" a language of provocation even when they are silent. We are no longer given verbal descriptions or exemplars of what a lady is or of what femininity consists. Rather we learn the rules directly through bodily discourse like images that tell us what clothes, body shape, facial expression, movements, and behavior are required. Indeed, aesthetics drive this image of the well-groomed eyebrow in modern cosmetic practice (Sadrô et al., 2003). Freund & Nolan (1996) revealed a correlation between brow life outcomes and aesthetic ideals for eyebrow height and shape in females. We believe that there is a close relationship between non-verbal eyebrow beauty and femininity. Evolutionary history has shown a considerable reduction in the amount of hair on the human face (McNeill, 2000). The presence of the eyebrows might seem a curiosity. Eyebrows give the eyes modest protection against such things as rain and perspiration; they have evolved and persisted owing to selection pressures associated, at least in part, with their role in facial attractiveness (Cosio & Robins, 2000), sexual dimorphism (Bruce et al., 1993), nonverbal communication and emotional expression (Ekman, 1979).

Practitioners in the field of facial aesthetics, such as make-up artists and cosmetic surgeons, have long appreciated the influence of the eyebrows on attractiveness (Cosio & Robins, 2000). During the 18th century in Western Europe, full eyebrows were in fact considered so essential to facial beauty that some upper-class women and courtiers would affix mouse hide to their foreheads. The perceived importance of the eyebrows in enhancing beauty has not waned to this day. Currently, it is relatively common cosmetic practice to use tweezers or depilatories to narrow and accentuate the arch of the eyebrows, as well as to remove any hair at the bridge of the nose. Cosmetics may also be used to alter the color, especially the darkness, and exaggerate the shape and length of the eyebrows. In addition, several cosmetic surgery procedures, including botulinum toxin, i.e. Botox injection (Huilgol et al., 2001), permanent tattooing, and surgical tucks and lifts, specifically target the appearance of the eyebrows (Sadrô et al., 2003).

Eyebrow tweezing and tattooing are very common practice in Hong Kong beauty salons, while coloring is not. This is because the color of Chinese eyebrows is already dark enough. It is likely that eyebrow surgery will become popular in the near future, given the increasing acceptance of cosmetic surgeries in Hong Kong.

Eyebrow tattooing is very common in Hong Kong and has been popular for almost twenty years. Tattooing equipment and techniques are continuously being developed and improved, demonstrating the huge demand for eyebrow beauty in Hong Kong, especially for women. The price ranges from several hundred to several thousand Hong Kong dollars per treatment. However, the price of eyebrow tattooing in mainland China is much lower than in Hong Kong, estimated at around RMB$300. People are therefore tempted to seek the treatment on the mainland, but this entails safety, hygiene and health risks. On the other hand, tattooing is seen as a "self-injury" (Inckle, 2005), which implies an internal psychological health risk. Bordo's (1993) idea highlighted the relationship between femininity and female beauty. We learn the importance of achieving "internal" women's health through "external" women's eyebrow beauty.

The global literature on the eyebrows addresses their anomalies (Waardenburg, 1951; Powell et al., 2001), their anatomy (Lemke & Stasior, 1982), the mechanism of eyebrow ptosis (Knize, 1996 a), eyebrow tumor (Boniuk & Zimmerman, 1972; Jho, 1997; Struijk et al., 2003), eyebrow lifting treatment (Connell, 1978; Gunter & Antrobus, 1997;

Knize, 1996 b), and reconstruction for burn patients (Burt, 1975; Sloan et al., 1976).

It is found in the literatures that different eyebrow movements or shapes are related to different facial expressions. Notably, the eyebrows were found to play a key role in the expression of a number of emotions (Ekman & Friesen, 1971; 1978; Ekman, 1993; 1979; Ellenbogen, 1983; Sadrô et al., 2003). Eyebrows A) inclined laterally transmit sadness; B) inclined medially transmit anger; C) lowered transmit tiredness; and D) properly aligned transmit an alert, rested countenance and allow the mouth to transmit the smile. On the other hand, seven experiments investigated the finding that threatening schematic faces are detected more quickly than nonthreatening faces (Tipples et al., 2002). Westmore presented a method of eyebrow shaping to establish a correct eyebrow in his makeup classes (Ellenbogen, 1983).

Alone, or in concert with other facial movements, changes in the angle, height, and curvature of the eyebrows can drastically alter the emotional expression of a face and may play an integral role in nonverbal communication. Closely related to the contribution of eyebrows to the facial expression of emotions is their involvement in other forms of communication. Previous work examining the functional role of eyebrow movements as conversational signals (e.g. Ekman, 1979), it is also interesting to observe the great extent to which the eyebrows are involved in purely nonverbal communication. An excellent demonstration of this comes from the domain of sign language (Baker-Shenk, 1985). Here, in the complete absence of vocal prosody, facial gestures (and eyebrow movements in particular) serve to modulate and complement that which has been signed by the hand and body. For example, raising the eyebrows quite naturally serves to recast a hand-signed expression as a question rather than a declarative statement, much in the same way that rising pitch can signal a question in a vocal utterance (Sadrô et al., 2003).

Apart from emotion, the eyebrows are also related to perception. Past work has examined the role of eyebrows in emotional expression and nonverbal communication, as well as in facial aesthetics and sexual dimorphism. Specifically, we find that the absence of eyebrows in familiar faces leads to a very large and significant disruption in recognition performance. In fact, a more significant decrease in face recognition is observed in the absence of eyebrows than in the absence of eyes (Sadrô et al., 2003).

One may expect the eyebrows to constitute an informative attribute for the task of face recognition. In one experiment, no-eyebrow and no-eye pictures of celebrities were constructed using computer software. Participants were asked to identify the celebrities. It was found that subjects were able to identify, on average, 30.1 of these 50 original images (SE=2.6. Consistent with previous reports, the absence of eyes significantly reduced subjects' ability to recognize the celebrities (mean=55.8%, SE=3.2%; $p<0.001$, paired t-test). In addition, however, the data revealed two other interesting results. First, with respect to the control condition, the celebrity images lacking eyebrows also proved remarkably difficult for subjects to identify (mean=46.3%, SE=4.4%; $p<0.001$). Second, recognition performance for faces without eyebrows was, in fact, significantly worse than that for faces without eyes (mean difference=9.5%, SE=4.8%; $p<0.05$). Surprisingly, therefore, face recognition appears to be disrupted even more by the absence of eyebrows than by the absence of eyes (Sadrô et al., 2003).

Nevertheless, in spite of the existing literature that has explored the involvement of eyebrows in such domains as facial aesthetics, gender discrimination, emotional expression, and nonverbal communication, the beauty treatments, treatment effects, reasons and health risks of eyebrow cosmetics have seldom been discussed.

## Eyebrow Beauty

Basically, eyebrow tweezing and trimming are always used to remove "chaotic" eyebrow hairs, so that a pair of neat eyebrows can give a clean image.

Besides eyebrow shaping, eyebrow designers usually lighten brows for clients because dark brows are heavy and can overpower all the other facial features. Turning down the depth of color a notch or two can bring them into balance. In the extreme, the eyebrows of a willing volunteer can be redrawn entirely after being physically 'erased' with cosmetic wax, sealer, and foundation (Aucoin, 1997).

Lightening brows is sometimes done but is not common for Chinese clients. Hong Kong women are more likely to seek darker brows or to fill in thin brows. This is not caused by a lack of eyebrow hair. Hair loss results from over-plucking and a low metabolism. Brows can be darkened by a simple eyebrow powder or cosmetic kits like stencils and wigs. Darker brows will be sharp and attractive, drawing the attention of others. However, eyebrow powders and cosmetic kits are not permanent. Impermanent eyebrows will come off in the pool, and even when sweating. Thus, permanent eyebrow tattooing is quite popular, as you can then forget about the brows. Certainly, there are disadvantages, in that there will be less choice in shape and color than with cosmetic makeup, and returns are difficult if you are not satisfied. Somehow, eyebrow shape is related to fashion trends. Different brow shapes can be made to match different fashions and images. Eyebrow tattooing should be carefully thought out before performing.

## Eyebrow Tattoo

As the shape of an eyebrow tattoo is difficult to change, a suitable eyebrow shape must be chosen before tattooing. According to the relationship between the eyebrows and facial expression, people choose eyebrow shapes in order to present different perceptions of themselves to others. In fact, the eyebrow shape should match the face shape as well. A simple example shows that a long face shape can look 'too long'. A flat eyebrow shape then shortens the face shape.

Freund & Nolan (1996) found a correlation between brow life outcomes and aesthetic ideals for eyebrow height and shape in females. Aesthetic criteria were determined by testing the opinions of 11 cosmetic surgeons and 9 cosmetologists. Eyebrow height and shape were altered with computer graphics to isolate those changes as the only variables of appearance. Three conclusions were drawn with regard to female eyebrows: (1) The medial eyebrow should be located at or below the supraorbital rim but not above it. (2) Eyebrow shape should have an apex lateral slant. (3) Standard open and endoscopic brow lift operations frequently result in unsatisfactory eyebrow height and shape, judged by these criteria. Although eyebrow beauty is usually sought by women, men have also started to care about their brows. Typically, a strong eyebrow, i.e. full, thick and massive, gives a stronger look. Powders and eyebrow gel are recommended to achieve this effect.

## DISCUSSION

Whatever the eyebrow beauty treatment, consumers should be aware of the chemical products. Heavy metals (Consumer Council, 1998) may be involved, and infections and inflammations (Consumer Council, 2001; Graves, 2000) can result. Especially with the eyebrow tattooing, bleeding commonly occurs, thus the needles and equipment used are always a concern. It is recommended that one-off, disposable needles be used, which should not be reused for another client even if sterilized because germs and diseases are easily transmitted when bleeding. However, reused needles are still very common in mainland China. This hygiene problem is of great concern. Two patients suffered epithelioid granulomatous inflammation of the eyebrows after undergoing cosmetic eyebrow tattooing. The causative elements were analyzed from biopsy specimens and tattoo inks with x-ray microanalysis. It is suggested that granuloma caused by cosmetic eyebrow tattooing is a complication worth mentioning (Yang et al., 1989). Problem color additives – Permanent Orange, Sudan II, Metanil Yellow, Scarlet Red, Methyl Violet BB, Gential Violet, Violet 6B and Rhodamine B – have been found in the dyes used in eyebrow beauty treatments. Some of these harmful substances are known to have caused cancer in rats and mice in laboratory experiments (Consumer Council, 1998). Taking proper care in the use of eyebrow beauty products is necessary to prevent infection and allow proper healing. All reputable eyebrow designers should give their clients detailed aftercare instructions.

More attention must be paid to eyebrow tattooing, as it involves the most health risks among all the eyebrow treatments. First, the color is difficult to remove, although it can now be removed with lasers. This is a relatively expensive procedure and is not totally successful. Sometimes it is impossible to regain the original skin color. Skin pigment can be lost and scarring often occurs. Government regulations should be established to prevent beauty treatment-related accidents. Muscle relaxation causes non-symmetrical eyebrows when aging (Lemke & Stasior, 1982). The lateral eyebrow has less support from deeper structures than the medial eyebrow, and the balance of forces acting on the eyebrow selectively depresses the lateral segment. Three forces that act on the lateral eyebrow are (1) the frontalis muscle resting tone, which suspends that eyebrow segment medial to the temporal fusion line of the skull, (2) gravity, which causes the soft-tissue mass lateral to the temporal line to slide over the temporalis fascia plane and push the lateral eyebrow segment downward, and (3) corrugator supercilii muscle hyperactivity in conjunction with the action of the lateral orbicularis oculi muscle, which can antagonize frontalis muscle activity and directly facilitate descent of the lateral eyebrow (Knize, 1996 a). Long ago, Castanares (1964) also indicated the relationship between the glabella frown and eyebrow ptosis. All the above factors may cause imperfect beauty. Serious consideration must be given to these factors before acquiring eyebrow tattoos.

It is observed that the majority of eyebrow-marked Hong Kong women re-mark their brows after a certain number of years, as the trend of eyebrow shapes changes, there are problems of symmetry, and the brow color fades. These reasons cause them to keep on tattooing. Another health risk, cosmetic addiction, is revealed as follows. In one case, a beautiful female aged twenty-five had less dense eyebrow hair. She used eyebrow powder every day in the past. Because of the inconvenience, she marked her brows. But she was unsatisfied even when the professional eyebrow designer felt her eyebrows were perfect. And she said that she thought she was prettier after each surgery. Finally her brows were tattooed three times by three different technicians in different shops within a month. In fact, the second tattoo should be done at least a month after the first. It was obvious that she was suffering from cosmetic addiction. It was recommended that she see a doctor.

It is not necessary to re-tattoo the eyebrows due to muscular relaxation. Radiofrequency application through a proprietary device has recently been used for facial tissue tightening. Using this technique, uniform volumetric heating of the dermis is created by the passage of an electrical current, while protection of the epidermis is maintained by concurrent cryogen cooling. Ten patients were treated on the left side of the face with radiofrequency, and changes in brow position, superior palpebral crease, angle of the eyebrow, and jowl surface area were evaluated in order to objectively quantify the effectiveness of volumetric radiofrequency application on the face. It was found that the application of radiofrequency to the face provides quantifiable changes. The brow along the midpupillary line is elevated to a greater degree than the lateral brow. This is consistent with the acute angle changes seen in the eyebrow (Nahm et al., 2004).

Modern techniques of micrograft hair transplantation can suitably re-create an aesthetic eyebrow in a case of iatrogenic eyebrow alopecia. Eyebrow transplantation is a suitable alternative to pedicle flap formation and composite scalp grafting. It is a straightforward procedure that can be performed in the office under local anesthesia with minimal attendant morbidity. The result may be superior to that seen with more involved eyebrow replacement procedures. Suitable aesthetic eyebrows were re-created in a symmetrical fashion with proper hair orientation. The process was time-consuming and tedious, but highly effective (Goldman, 2001).

## IMPLICATIONS

Psychological health risk has an equally important association with the physical health risks of eyebrow beauty. An eyebrow tattoo can be seen as a "self-injury" (Inckle, 2005). Modification can offer women a means of 'control, stability, and empowerment' and allow them 'to overcome the oppressive potentialities that the female has through her own body'. Most women in our culture, then, are somehow "disordered" when it comes to issues of self-worth, self-entitlement, self-nourishment, and comfort with their own bodies. Our culture has not only taught women to be insecure bodies, constantly monitoring themselves for signs of imperfection, constantly engaged in physical "improvement"; it is also constantly teaching women how to see their bodies.

A definition of the feminine concept can be found in Bordo (1993). Beauty and sexuality can function as a medium of power and control for the otherwise powerless. Social manipulation of the female body has emerged as an absolutely central strategy in the maintenance of power relations between the sexes over the past hundred years. Through beauty modification, women can feel their own femininity. Eyebrows play an important role in human face recognition (Duda et al., 2001; Sadrô et al., 2003). These authors also suggest that darker brows are sharper and more attractive, drawing the attention of others. The eyebrows and the feminine self they symbolize are a vital part of who they are.

Females increase their "normalizing power" through the "pathological method" to meet the standard of the beauty culture so that they are then ideal in terms of power, will, mastery, and the possibilities of success in the professional arena. Otherwise, failure will be perceived as indicative of laziness, lack of discipline, unwillingness to conform and absence of all those "managerial" abilities that, according to the dominant ideology, confer upward mobility. This preoccupation with the "internal" management of the body (that is, management of its desires) is produced by instabilities in what could be called the macro-regulation of desire within the system of the social body.

Another example is slenderness: most women, regardless of their socioeconomic class, are affected by the "tenacious and all-pervasive" ideal of the perfect feminine figure. These associations are carried visually by the slender superwomen of prime time television and popular movies, and promoted explicitly in advertisements and articles appearing routinely in women's fashion magazines, diet books, and weight training publications. Yet the thousands of slender girls and women who strive to embody these images, and who in that service suffer from eating disorders, exercise compulsions, and continual self-scrutiny and self-castigation, are anything but the "masters" of their lives. Popular representations, as we have seen, may forcefully employ the rhetoric and symbolism of empowerment, personal freedom, having it all. Yet female bodies, pursuing these ideals, may find themselves as distracted, depressed, and physically ill as female bodies in the nineteenth century became when pursuing a feminine ideal of dependency, domesticity and delicacy.

It should be noted that while cosmetic tattooing has a psychological benefit to the person, the same reasoning might be applied to a person with a personality disorder characterized by developmental defects or pathological trends in the personality structure with minimal subjective anxiety, giving a certain psychological benefit from tattooing (Post, 1968). Many "self-injury" treatments are very popular in the beauty industry. There is still much room for exploration of the psychological reasons behind this popularity. The work of this article is merely pioneering, intended to raise awareness. It is hoped that further and more in-depth studies can be carried out, and that other researchers will contribute more to the field of beauty and health for better health promotion and education for women.

## CONCLUSION

Eyebrow beauty treatments, especially eyebrow tattoos, are popular among Hong Kong women. However, this cosmetic topic and the associated health risks are seldom discussed. The eyebrows are related to facial aesthetics, gender discrimination, emotional expression, and nonverbal communication. Different eyebrow shapes can give different impressions and images. There is also evidence that eyebrows play an important role in human face recognition and attract attention from others. All these factors support the pursuit of eyebrow beauty. However, the chemical, hygiene, and accidental problems that affect consumers' health must be addressed. Government legislation can play an important role in such regulation. In this article, I have argued that the availability of female beauty signifies a sense of hope that femininity and instability can be balanced, which in turn will enable a harmony to exist between body and self. The addiction and "self-injury" psychological angles can also be further studied for better women's health promotion and education.

# REFERENCES

Aucoin, K. (1997). *Making Faces*. Boston, MA: Little, Brown and Co.

Baker-Shenk, C. (1985). The facial behavior of deaf signers: Evidence of a complex language. *American Annals of the Deaf, 130*,297-304.

Boniuk, M., & Zimmerman, L.E. (1972). Sebaceous Carcinoma of the Eyelid, Eyebrow, Caruncle, and Orbit. *Spring, 12*(1),225-257.

Bordo, S. (1993). *Unbearable Weight, Feminism, Western Culture and The Body*. Berkeley: University of California Press.

Bruce, V., Burton, A.M., Hanna, E., Healey, P., Mason, O., Coombes, A., Fright, R., & Linney, A. (1993). Sex discrimination: how do we tell the difference between male and female faces? *Perception, 22*,131-152.

Burt, B. (1975). Reconstruction of ear, eyebrow, and sideburn in the burned patient. *Plastic and Reconstructive Surgery, 55*(3),312-317.

Castanares, S. (1964). Forehead Wrinkles, Glabellar Frown and Ptosis of the Eyebrows. *Plastic and Reconstructive Surgery, 34*(4),406-413.

Connell, B.F. (1978). Eyebrow, face, and neck lifts for males. *Clin Plast Surg, 5*(1),15-28.

Consumer Council. (1998). Press Releases: Clean bill of health for color cosmetics. Retrieved February 08, 2010, from http://www.consumer. org.hk/website/ws_en/news/press_releases/p261.html

Consumer Council. (2001). Press Releases: Beauty and slimming centers in consumer complaints over unethical and misleading practices. Retrieved February 08, 2010, from http://www.consumer.org.hk /website/ws_en/news/press_releases/p295.html

Cosio, R., & Robins, C. (2000). *The Eyebrow*. New York: Harper Collins.

Duda, R. O., Hart, P.E., & Stork, D.G. (2001). *Pattern Classification.* (2nd ed.). New York: John Wiley.

Ekman, P., & Friesen, W.V. (1971). Constants across cultures in the face and emotion. *Journal of Personality and Social Psychology, 17,*124-129.

Ekman, P., & Friesen, W.V. (1978). *Facial Action Coding System.* Palo Alto, CA: Consulting Psychologists Press.

Ekman, P. (1979). About brows: Emotional and conversational signals. In M. Von Cranach, K. Foppa, W. Lepenies, & D. Ploog (eds.), *Human Ethology: Claims and Limits of a New Discipline* (pp. 169-202). Cambridge: Cambridge University Press.

Ekman, P. (1993). Facial expression of emotion. *American Psychologist, 48,*384-392.

Ellenbogen, R. (1983). Transcoronal Eyebrow Lift with Concomitant Upper Blepharoplasty. *Plastic and Reconstructive Surgery, 71*(4),490-499.

Freund, R.M., & Nolan, W.B. (1996). Correlation Between Brow Life Outcomes and Aesthetic Ideals for Eyebrow Height and Shape in Females. *Plastic & Reconstructive Surgery, 97*(7),1343-1348.

Goldman, G.D. (2001). Eyebrow Transplantation. *Dermatologic Surgery, 27*(4),352-354.

Graves, B.B. (2000). *Tattooing and Body Piercing.* Capstone Press.

Gunter, J.P., & Antrobus, S.D. (1997). Aesthetic Analysis of the Eyebrows. *Plastic & Reconstructive Surgery, 99*(7),1808-1816.

Huck, V. (1998). *The adorned and the ambivalent.* Staffordshire, UK: Keele University Press.

Huilgol, S.C., Carruthers, A., & Carruthers, J.D.A. (2001). Raising Eyebrows with Botulinum Toxin. *Dermatologic Surgery, 25*(5),373-376.

Inckle, K. (2005). Who's Hurting Who? The Ethics of Engaging the Marked Body. *Auto/Biography, 13,*227-248.

Jho, H.D. (1997). Orbital Roof Craniotomy Via an Eyebrow Incision: A Simplified Anterior Skull Base Approach. *Thieme, 40*(3),91-97.

Knize, D.M. (1996 a). An Anatomically Based Study of the Mechanism of Eyebrow Ptosis. *Journal of the American Society of Plastic Surgeon, 97*(7),1321-1333.

Knize, D.M. (1996 b). Limited-Incision Forehead Lift for Eyebrow Elevation to Enhance Upper Blepharoplasty. *Plastic & Reconstructive Surgery, 97*(7),1334-1342.

Lemke, B.N., & Stasior, O.G. (1982). The Anatomy of Eyebrow Ptosis. *Arch Ophthalmol, 100*(6),981-986.

McNeill, D. (2000). *The Face: A Natural History*. Boston, MA: Little, Brown and Co.

Nahm, W.K., Su, T.T., Rotunda, A.M., & Moy, R.L. (2004). Objective Changes in Brow Position, Superior Palpebral Crease, Peak Angle of the Eyebrow, and Jowl Surface Area after Volumetric Radiofrequency Treatments to Half of the Face. *Dermatologic Surgery, 30*(6),922-928.

Post, R.S. (1968). The relationship of tattoos to personality disorders. *The Journals of Criminal Law, Criminology & Police Sciences, 59*(4).

Powell, J., Dawber, R.P.R., & Ferguson, D.J.P. (2001). Netherton's syndrome: increased likelihood of diagnosis by examining eyebrow hairs. *British Journal of Dermatology, 141*(3),544-546.

Sadrô, J., Jarudi, I., & Sinhaô, P. (2003). The role of eyebrows in face recognition. *Perception, 32*,285-293.

Sloan, D.F., Huang, T.T., Larson, D.L., & Lewis, S.R. (1976). Reconstruction of Eyelids and Eyebrows in Burned Patients. *Plastic and Reconstructive Surgery, 58*(3),340-346.

Struijk, L., Bavinck, J.N.B., Wanningen, P., Meijden, E.V., Westendorp, R.G.J., Schegget, J.T., & Feltkamp, M.C.W. (2003). Presence of Human Papillomavirus DNA in Plucked Eyebrow Hairs Is Associated with a History of Cutaneous Squamous Cell Carcinoma. *Journal of Investigative Dermatology, 121*,1531-1535.

Tipples, J., Atkinson, A.P., & Young, A.W. (2002). The eyebrow frown: A salient social signal. *Emotion, 2*(3),288-296.

Waardenburg, P.J. (1951). A new syndrome combining developmental anomalies of the eyelids, eyebrows and noseroot with pigmentary anomalies of the iris and head hair and with congenital deafness; Dystopia canthi medialis et punctorum lacrimalium lateroversa, hyperplasia supercilii medialis et radicis nasi, heterochromia iridum totaliis sive partialis, albinismus circumscriptus (leucismus, polioss) et surditas congenita (surdimutitas). *Am J Hum Genet, 3*(3),195-253.

Yang, D.S., Kim, S.C., Lee, S., & Chung, Y. (1989). Foreign body epithelioid granuloma after cosmetic eyebrow tattooing. *Cutis, 43*(3), 244-247.

# Chapter 4

# NAIL BEAUTY AND HEALTH

## *Zenobia C. Y. Chan and Queeni T. Y. Ip*
The Hong Kong Polytechnic University, China

## ABSTRACT

Nail care should be seen as personal hygiene, but beautiful nails are perceived as a representation of feminine beauty. Recently, artificial fingernails have become very popular in Hong Kong. Chemical gels coat the nail surface for artificial nail extensions. Chemicals are known to be harmful to our health. However, Hong Kong women continue to seek nail beauty. A lack of literature about nail beauty and women's health in Hong Kong and elsewhere has been found. This paper explores how nail beauty therapy affects Hong Kong women and how their nail beauty affects their psychological well-being. It suggests that psychological health risks including perfectionism, failure and addiction might be behind the nail beauty industry, which can be explained by the objectification theory. We foresee that a by-product, sexual objectification, is emerging from the self-objectification. The phenomenon of "lewd young model" is emerging in Hong Kong. This objectification of women may influence the thinking of the younger generation and affect their social health. This paper aims to reveal some of the implications for health education.

# INTRODUCTION

## History of Nail Beauty

In the past, nail beauty therapy was used as a status symbol, indicating that, unlike commoners, the nail owner was not accustomed to doing manual labor. In the late 20th century, artificial nails for women have become popular all over the world. Nail beauty in various countries will be reviewed in this section. Noblewomen in China's Ming Dynasty wore long artificial nails. The Chinese used a colored lacquer made from a combination of Arabic gum, egg whites, gelatin and beeswax. They also used a mixture consisting of mashed rose, orchid and impatiens petals, combined with alum. A pink to red color resulted after leaving such mixtures on the nails for a few hours or overnight. Royalty used gold and silver to enhance their nails in the Chou Dynasty. A Ming manuscript also cites red and black as the colors chosen by royalty.

Egyptians used reddish-brown stains derived from henna to color their nails. They used nail color to signify social order, with shades of red at the top. Queen Nefertiti colored her finger and toe nails ruby red, while Cleopatra favored a deep rust red. Women of lower rank who colored their nails were permitted only pale hues. On the other hand, Americans had colorful nails too. It is unclear how the practice of coloring nails progressed following these beginnings. Portraits from the 17th and 18th centuries include shiny nails. In the 19th century, nails were tinted with scented red oils and polished or buffed with a chamois cloth, rather than simply painted. In addition, 19th century cookbooks in England and the United States contained directions for making nail paints. In the 19th and early 20th centuries, women still pursued a polished, rather than painted, look by massaging tinted powders and creams into their nails, then buffing them shiny. One such polishing product sold around this time was Graf's Hyglo nail polish paste. Some women during this period painted their nails using a clear, glossy varnish applied with camel-hair brushes. When automobile paint was created in around 1920, it inspired the introduction of colored nail enamels. Nail polish contains nitrocellulose, which is available in many different grades and is measured by viscosity.

From the above various perceptions and strategies regarding nail beauty, it seems that nails are a significant body part in expressing women's beauty desire. The next section presents some of the current views on nail beauty.


## Current Views of Nail Beauty

The tradition of nail beauty started a long time ago and is generally seen as part of personal beauty and care. Nail beauty therapy is usually followed by hand treatment. A common type of manicure involves shaping the nails and applying nail polish. Artificial nails have been found in manicures more recently. Some manicures can include the painting of pictures or designs on the nails, or applying small decals or imitation jewels. Some artificial nails attempt to mimic the look of real fingernails, while other designs may deliberately stray in look from real fingernails. A nail technician specializes in the art form and care of nails, including manicures, pedicures, acrylic nails, gel nails, nail wraps, fake nails, etc. Special techniques can be used for those who are allergic to chemicals. Nail technicians are also knowledgeable in nail irregularities and diseases, and may be able to identify such problems. They do not treat diseases and typically refer a client to a physician if the need arises. There are also temporary, cheaper, and flexible tips that can be quickly glued on at home without help from a professional.


## Nail Beauty in Hong Kong

Many organizations and schools, including the Vocational Education Training Council, provide nail art courses (VTC, 2009). In addition, 19 inmates of the Lai Chi Kok Correctional Institution (LCKCI) received professional nail therapist certificates in programs designed as part of a rehabilitation project for prisoners, jointly organized by the Hong Kong Correctional Services and the Hong Kong Hair and Beauty Merchants Association (GovHK, 2007). The potential development of nail beauty therapy in Hong Kong can be seen. On the other hand, Michael Kalow, chairman of the German-based Wilde Cosmetics, one of the world's largest manufacturers of nail, hand and foot care products in the world, said his company is committed to expanding its presence in Asia, and Hong Kong was the company's first choice for its regional headquarters (GovHK, 2005). This indicates that Hong Kong and Asia represent a huge potential future nail market. According to the 2003 manpower survey tables by the beauty care and hairdressing training board of the Vocational Training Council, manicurists, pedicurists and nail artists are usually distributed in beauty care centers, makeup and nail schools, hairdressing salons, health centers and spas (VTC, 2003). Based on the population census of 2007, there are as many as 27,000 frontline staff and 8,000 shops in this industry.

The principal of the Caritas Cosmetic Career Center, Ms. Leung, said that each frontline member of staff should have several different professional beauty skills and techniques by now, with no more focusing on one skill as in the beauty industry in the past (JUMP, 2009). Besides, as Ms. Janice Chan, Education Manager from Sheer Nail of IL COLPO Group, pointed out, male manicurists or pedicurists and male customers are to be found more recently (JiuJik, 2007). Also, as the director of Creation Nail Professional said, customers' demands are no longer for a manicure only; they need more skillful techniques and knowledge, for example, gel extension and 3D nail art. Frontline staff should get professional certification, says a Local or Overseas Professional Training Course Certificate (JUMP, 2009). As for the market price of nail beauty therapy, it ranges from one to several hundred Hong Kong dollars, depending on the different techniques, products and accessories used.

In Hong Kong, discussions of nails are usually about careers, products and courses, but few mention the relationship between nail beauty and health for Hong Kong women, even though it is already a visible beauty trend, common and popular. In fact, there are known and hidden health risks behind nail beauty. This paper explores the experiences of Hong

Kong women with regard to nail beauty. It then discusses how nail beauty affects Hong Kong women's psychological health. Finally, it aims to draw some implications for health education and behavior regarding this underexplored female health issue.

## LITERATURE REVIEW

Global literature about nails usually talks about medical (Zaias, 1990), physical (Baden, 1970), chemical (Houlihan & Wiles, 2000), disease (Geyer et al., 2004), and histological issues (Suarez et al., 1991), as well as fungus, etiology and treatment (Baran & Haneke, 2004), potential hazards (Baran, 2002b), and allergies and irritations (Baran, 2002a). For example, the harmful effects of nail polish are always a hot topic. OPI Nail Products, a leading producer of professional nail care products, offers safer versions for the European market, but not for U.S. consumers, and has refused to replace the toxic ingredients that are linked to cancer and birth defects (Pitman, 2006a). On the other hand, another major nail varnish manufacturer said they would remove chemicals linked to cancer and birth defects from their formulations. However, the company has not yet confirmed when all the reformulated products will be on store shelves. Both OPI and Orly said they would remove DBP from their products but would continue to use toluene. Likewise, OPI still uses formaldehyde in some nail products. Orly spokesperson Jennifer Marlowe said that the company began removing DBP from all products "at least a year ago", but that "some products still contain small amounts of toluene and formaldehyde resin, not formaldehyde".

In fact, three ingredients are on California's Prop. 65 list of chemicals known to cause cancer or reproductive toxicity. In particular, recent scientific studies have stressed the link between DBP and the underdevelopment of newborn baby boys. Although the chemical is banned by the European Union, the U.S. FDA has not made any such move. Toluene has also been linked to skin irritations, liver damage and anemia, while formaldehyde is 'reasonably anticipated' to be a human carcinogen. The group says that its action against specific manufacturers of nail varnish highlights the fact that FDA regulations do not require that cosmetics products be tested for safety, contrary to stricter regulations governing the European market. Fortunately, Avon, Estee Lauder, Revlon and L'Oreal have already confirmed that they will remove DBP from their nail varnish formulations (Pitman, 2006b).

Besides the DBP, phthalates from nail varnish are considered in the US to be potentially dangerous substances. Scientific studies have in the past shown a link between the presence of phthalates during pregnancy and the low birth weight of infants and breast cancer. Phthalates are commonly used in cosmetic and personal care products such as hairspray, nail varnish and fragrance (Harrington & Pitman, 2009). In addition, scientists in northern France have carried out a comprehensive study encompassing 3,421 women to determine the effects of occupational exposure to solvents while pregnant in a range of occupations including beauticians, hairdressers, nurses, chemists and biologists. Hairdressers and beauticians are exposed to a variety of solvents in beauty products, but most commonly those from hairspray and hairstyling products, as well as solvents used in nail varnish. The scientists found that the level of exposure to solvents while pregnant, when compared with the rate of congenital malformations, showed a clear pattern of increased risk of problems. Likewise, the results showed that the risk of problems such as oral clefts, urinary malformations and male genital malformations, increased in direct correlation with the level of exposure to solvents in pregnant working women from specific subgroups in the study. The scientists said that the conclusion of their study clearly points to a correlation between exposure to solvents while pregnant and the risk of major malformations (Pitman, 2009).

In fact, there is evidence that chemicals used in nail beauty therapy do have harmful effects on human health. However, women are still enjoying nail beauty for themselves. Therefore, this chapter will present the real cases of Hong Kong women who tried nail beauty even with knowledge of its potential harm, and aims to explore the psychological reasons for the desire for nail beauty and study how nail beauty affects Hong Kong women's health.

There is a lack of global literature on the psychological approach to nail beauty therapy. Additionally, literature about nail beauty for women and how nail beauty therapy affects women's psychological health is seldom found. To fill the above gaps, we will present some case studies observed by the second author, who is a beauty therapist with experience of providing nail beauty for women from various backgrounds in Hong Kong.

## CASE STUDIES

It is rare that Hong Kong women seek nail beauty therapy to cover up problematic nails. Interestingly, the main reason for pursuing nail beauty therapy is the desire for "perfect beauty", although they understand that it entails certain harms before they embark upon such therapy. Four case studies will be illustrated.

### Case 1 - Nail Shape Improvement

Amy Wong, 21 years old, is a fresh graduate. She is looking for a clerical job. However, her nails are rotten. This is not good for her interviews. So she got simple artificial nails, not in the exaggerated style. She requested a mere improvement in her nail shape, not the long nail extensions. She said: "I would like to give a holistic, clean, healthy and practical image to potential employers. I don't want my rotten nails to give them an impression of carelessness."

## Case 2 - Non-yellowing of the nails

Sandy Lai, 49 years old, is a housewife. She has practiced nail beauty for ten years. In the past, she used to use nail polish only. However, recently she is really enjoying artificial nails. She says: "The gel coating can prevent the nail enamel from coming into direct contact with the nail surface. The gel does not make the surface of my nails yellow. I feel that my nails are healthier and prettier even when they are naked." She also said: "The edges of my nails are thick, not sharp enough to cut me and leave scars on my skin, even if I have long extensions."

Although the nail enamel does not come into direct contact with the nail surface, this does not mean that there are no chemicals on the nail surface. Chemicals contain nylon fibers, acrylate resin and hydrolyzed proteins. Others may contain up to 5% formaldehyde tissue fixative (Baran, 2002a).

## Case 3 - Frontline Staff

Sou Ip, 28 years old, is a member of frontline staff in the service industry. She has all healthy nails but still seeks nail beauty therapy continuously as she wants to beautify every part of her body. She says: "Customers see my hands every day; they look at my hands when I give them their change. Charming nails can draw attention from others. They are the second most important thing following a pair of young and delicate hands. Nail beauty can make me more attractive."

## Case 4 - Bridal

May Lee, 29 years old, is getting married. She has put nothing on her nails in the past but has tried artificial nails twice: once for the wedding photos and once for her wedding party. She said: "I want to be a beautiful and perfect bride: facial and slimming treatments, nail beauty therapy and hair removal should all be done well for my big day, so I will try nail beauty even though I think it is quite inconvenient with the extended nails."

From the above four cases, a common reason for nail beauty therapy is the pursuit of better and perfect beauty. All hoped to create a positive image for others. People seldom seek nail beauty therapy because of disease and infection. Conversely, it was observed that they would stop nail beauty therapy if they found something wrong with their nails. Although nail beauty therapy can make the nails look attractive, it masks our health risks, as we cannot observe emerging problems if our nails are masked by a coating.

## DISCUSSION

The above cases show the reasons why Hong Kong women seek nail beauty. The most common reason is that they want to create a positive image and attract attention from others with their charming and attractive nails, even though there are disadvantages to nail beauty. Some examples of these are chemical absorption from nail varnish, yellowing of the nail surfaces when naked, nail varnish easily fading after several washes, contamination when cooking, transfer of contamination to children, nail infections (Baran, 2002b), skin allergies and irritation (Baran, 2002a), and abrasion to cause a thinner nail surface.

For these reasons, artificial nails are becoming popular because they still have benefits, but with fewer risks. Artificial nails help to conceal or fix broken, damaged, short, or bad nails. They also help to prevent people from biting and breaking their nails, and protect nails from splitting. They are used when people are not able to grow the length and strength of natural nails that they desire. Besides the physical benefits, a psychological analysis of nail beauty should be conducted.

## Psychological Perspectives on Nail Beauty

For Case 1, Amy would like to give a positive image to others, rather than letting them see her rotten nails. This is because women seem to be afraid of letting others see how they really are (Chrisler, 2008). In Case 2, Sandy is looking for a healthier nail. It is easy to understand that people try to do the best they can (Chrisler, 2008).

When people try to achieve their personal best, it can be seen as chasing standards, both internally and externally. However, the internalized standards for women are often unrealistic, even though they are thought to be ideal (Chrisler, 2008). Perfectionism can be seen in the above four cases, especially Case 4. Saltzberg and Chrisler (1995) indicated that ideals can only be achieved by a small group. If too many people get close to an ideal, it will have to change in order to maintain its extraordinary nature.

Although nail beauty can have a positive psychological effect on women, it is also dangerous and harms their psychological health. It is believed that our culture encourages us to strive for the ideal (Chrisler, 2008). Case 3 showed that attractive nails are part of the beauty culture. People agree that artificial nails are beautiful. Sou is seeking agreement with others. These cultural demands that women pursue beauty have been described as oppressive and dangerous (Dworkin, 1974). When beauty ideals change, women's bodies are expected to change too (Saltzberg & Chrisler, 1995). This ideal is unnatural and impossible to achieve, so failure and sadness will be the eventual result (Freedman, 1988).

It is curious that women are out of control if they do not approach beauty ideals. Questions must be asked about what is behind this ideal of perfectionism. Hong Kong women are influenced by western education and culture. American culture encourages people to control their lives (Brownell, 1991; McDaniel, 1988; Ussher, 2004). And the image of the superwoman has already been well developed in Hong Kong. Both these images require perfectionism. A perfectionist is a person who sets rigid, unrealistically high standards and engages in "all-or-nothing" thinking when evaluating her performance (Campbell & DiPaula, 2002). There is a very high risk that anything that is not perfect will be a failure. Perfectionism has been associated with eating disorders (Forbush et al., 2007) and excessive exercise (Shroff et al., 2006), as well as with stress, anger, anxiety and depression (Antony & Swinson, 1988; Frost & DiBartolo, 2002; Hewitt & Flett 1991, 1993).

As we explained above, the theory behind this ideal of perfectionism is objectification. Objectification theory is based on the principle that girls and women develop their primary view of their physical selves from observations of others through the media or personal experience (Bartky, 1990). Females are socialized to self-objectify their own physical characteristics from a third person perspective (Kaschak, 1992). Interestingly, they are aware that others are likely to observe them as well, apart from the observations of others. Objectification theory is essential in feminist theory, as the sexual objectification and self-objectification of women is believed to influence social gender roles and inequalities between the sexes (Goldenberg & Tomi-Ann, 2004).

Self-objectification increases the awareness of an individual's physical appearance (Fredrickson & Kristen, 2005). When individuals know that others are looking at them, or will be looking at them, they are more likely to care about their physical appearance. Women's bodies are often objectified and evaluated more frequently (Fredrickson & Kristen, 2005). Females learn that their physical appearance is important both to themselves and society. As a result, females consider their physical appearance often and expect that others will do likewise.

Sexual objectification occurs when a person is identified by their sexual body parts or sexual function. In essence, an individual loses their identity and is recognized solely by the physical characteristics of their body (Bartky, 1990). The purpose of this recognition is to bring enjoyment to others, or to serve as a sexual object for society (LeMoncheck, 1997). Sexual objectification may have resulted from placing too much emphasis on self-objectification.

We have learned that objectification theory is valuable to understanding how repeated visual images in the media are socialized and translated into mental health problems, including psychological consequences at the individual and societal levels (Fredrickson & Tomi-Ann, 1997). We believe that self-consciousness, body anxiety, mental health threats and body shame will be increased (Fredrickson & Tomi-Ann, 1997; Fredrickson & Kristen, 2005). The effects of objectification theory are identified at both the individual and societal levels.

Feminist Ariel Levy contends that Western women have begun to sexually objectify themselves by choice, by wearing increasingly revealing clothing and engaging in lewd behavior. Sometimes it is seen as empowerment, although critics contend that it has led to greater emphasis on women's perceived self-worth (Parker, 2008). Levy argues that contemporary America's sexualized culture not only objectifies women but also encourages them to objectify themselves (Dougary, 2007). We question whether this new "raunchy" culture marked not the ruin of feminism but its triumph in winning women's right to express their sexuality publicly. A similar situation in the form of the lewd young model issue is emerging in Hong Kong. Health education should be targeted at preventing the deterioration of feminism and social health (Figure 1).

Although there are as yet no data related to nail beauty therapy and psychological health for Hong Kong women, many related physical and psychological health issues should be examined in the future. I hope this article will give a fresh insight into the psychological health aspect of beauty, which is closely related to women's health in general.

An ideal should be admired, while excellence should be that for which we strive (Chrisler, 2008). In fact, nail therapy has health benefits for people. However, continuous nail beauty therapy may, like cosmetic surgery, cause a beauty addiction that is not recommended. There are still many toxins contained in the coatings. Environmental Protection Agency (EPA) chief Lisa Jackson says that the Agency has inadequate tools to protect against chemical risks, and the public is understandably anxious and confused as the presence of chemicals has become ubiquitous in our environment and our bodies (Harrington & Pitman, 2009). Labeling and legislation issues should also be addressed in health promotion and education.

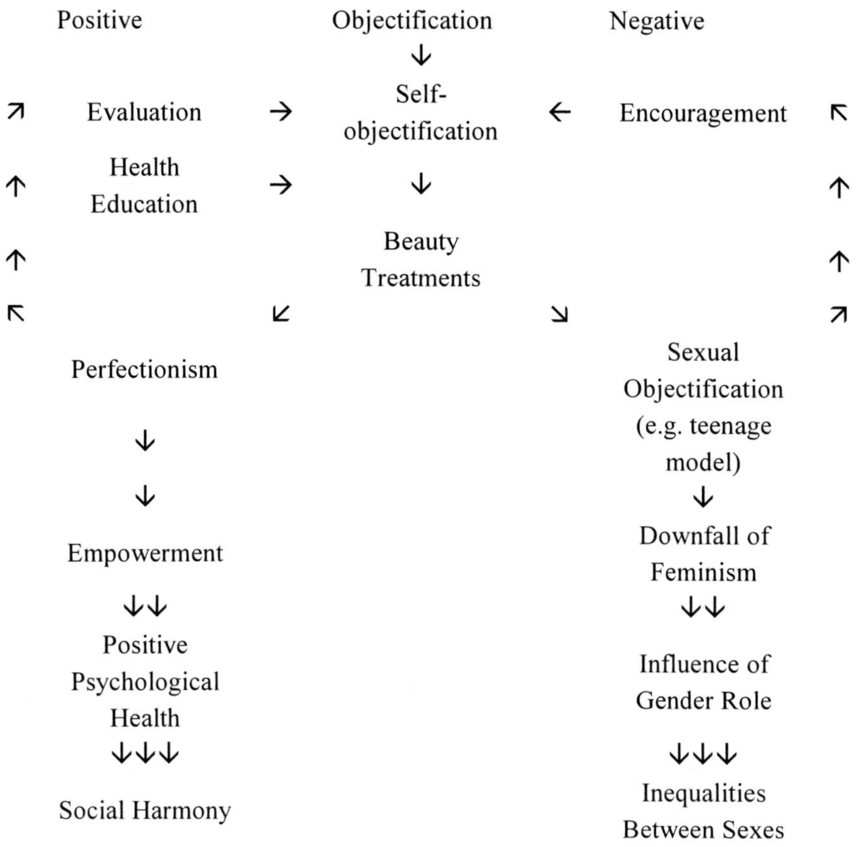

| Positive | | Objectification | | Negative | |
|---|---|---|---|---|---|
| | | ↓ | | | |
| ↗ | Evaluation | → | Self-objectification | ← Encouragement | ↖ |
| ↑ | Health Education | → | ↓ | | ↑ |
| ↑ | | | Beauty Treatments | | ↑ |
| ↖ | | ↙ | | ↘ | ↗ |
| | Perfectionism | | | Sexual Objectification (e.g. teenage model) | |
| | ↓ | | | ↓ | |
| | ↓ | | | Downfall of Feminism | |
| | Empowerment | | | ↓↓ | |
| | ↓↓ | | | Influence of Gender Role | |
| | Positive Psychological Health | | | ↓↓↓ | |
| | ↓↓↓ | | | Inequalities Between Sexes | |
| | Social Harmony | | | | |

Figure 1. The relationship of health education to beauty treatment and feminism.

## New Trends in Nail Beauty

Owing to the harmful effects of nail therapy, a new trend can be observed in nail beauty in Hong Kong: Calgel. Calgel is a new nail product, the result of scientific development, that is bringing many advantages to nail therapy (Calgel USA, Inc., 2008). The main difference compared to the traditional artificial nail is that it will not inhibit natural metabolic activity, and will allow natural nails to breathe. In addition, Katie Bird suggests that nail varnish that can be switched on or off, and environmentally-friendly pigments such as iron oxide, which can instantly and reversibly change color, could be the future of color cosmetics. Magnetic fields act externally on the orientation of these microspheres without changing the structure of the microspheres themselves, according to researchers in California (Bird, 2009). It is expected that if the industry is able to produce environmentally friendly and scientific beauty products, this will have a positive impact on the public in the future.

## CONCLUSION

The presented cases suggest that Hong Kong women like to draw attention from others by using nail beauty therapy to obtain attractive nails and present a healthy and perfect image to the world. However, common artificial nails cause certain harm to nails. Although they may have psychological benefits for these women, they also cause potential psychological harm at an individual and societal level. It is recommended that women balance their psychological health with their nail health, and it is hoped that scientific work and nail product manufacturers will begin to provide less harmful products so as to protect the health of this small but important area of the body.

## REFERENCES

Antony, M.M., & Swinson, R.P. (1998). *When perfect isn't good enough: Strategies for coping with perfectionism.* New York: Barnes & Noble/ New Harbinger.

Baden, H.P. (1970). The physical properties of nail. *Journal of Investigative Dermatology, 55,*115-122.

Baran, R. (2002a). Nail Cosmetics: Allergies and Irritations. *American Journal of Clinical Dermatology, 3,*547-555.

Baran, R. (2002b). Nail beauty therapy: an attractive enhancement or a potential hazard? *Journal of Cosmetic Dermatology, 1,*24-29.

Baran, R., & Haneke, M. (2004). Etiology and Treatment of Nail Malalignment. *Dermatologic Surgery, 24,*719-721.

Bartky, S.L. (1990). Femininity and Domination: Studies in the Phenomenology of Oppression. Routledge.

Bird, K. (2009). Nail varnish that can be switched on or off: The future of color cosmetics? Retrieved October 9, 2009, from http://www. cosmeticsdesign.com/Product-Categories/Color-Cosmetics/Nail-varnish-that-can-be-switched-on-or-off-The-future-of-color-cosmetics

Brownell, K. (1991). Personal responsibility and control over our bodies: When expectation exceeds reality. *Health Psychology, 10,*303-310.

Calgel USA, Inc. (2008). Why Calgel? Retrieved September 19, 2009, from http://www.calgelusa.com/whycalgel.htm

Campbell, J.D., & DiPaula, A. (2002). Perfectionistic self-beliefs: Their relation to personality and goal pursuit. In G.L.Flett & P.L.Hewitt (eds.), *Perfectionism: Theory, research, and treatment* (pp.181-198). Washington, DC: American Psychological Association.

Chrisler, J.C. (2008). 2007 Presidential address: Fear of losing control: Power, perfectionism, and the psychology of women. *Psychology of Women Quarterly, 32,*1-12.

Dougary, G. (2007). "Yes we are bovvered". Retrieved May 23, 2010, from http://women.timesonline.co.uk/tol/life_and_style/women/ article 523264.ece

Dworkin, A. (1974). *Woman hating.* New York: Dutton.

Fredrickson, B.L., & Kristen, H. (2005). Throwing like a girl: Self-objectification predicts adolescent girl's motor performance. *Journal of Sport and Social Issues, 29,*79-101.

Fredrickson, B.L., & Tomi-Ann, R. (1997). Objectification Theory: Toward understanding women's lived experiences and mental health risks. *Psychology of Women Quarterly, 21,*173-206.

Freedman, R. (1988). Bodylove: Learning to like our looks – and ourselves. New York: Harper & Row.

Frost, R.O., & DiBartolo, P.M. (2002). Perfectionism, anxiety, and obsessive-compulsive disorder. In G.L.Flett & P.L.Hewitt (eds.),

*Perfectionism: Theory, research, and treatment* (pp. 341-371). Washington, DC: American Psychological Association.

Forbush, K., Heatherton, T.F., & Keel, P.K. (2007). Relationships between perfectionism and specific disordered eating behaviors. *International Journal of Eating Disorders, 40,*37-41.

Geyer, A., Onumah, N., Uyttendaele, H., & Scher, R. (2004). Modulation of linear nail growth to treat diseases of the nail. *Journal of the American Academy of Dermatology, 50,*229-234.

Goldenberg, J.L., & Tomi-Ann, R. (2004). The beast within the beauty: An existential perspective on the objectification and condemnation of women. In J.Greenberg, S.L.Koole & T.Pyszczynski (eds.), *Handbook of experimental existential psychology* (pp. 71-85). Guilford Press.

GovHK. (2005). Press Release: German cosmetics group forms JV in Hong Kong as Asia-Pacific base. Retrieved October 7, 2009, from http://www.info.gov.hk/gia/general/200503/16/03160084.htm

GovHK. (2007). Press Release: LCKCI inmates receive professional nail therapist certificates. Retrieved October 7, 2009, from http://www.info. gov .hk/gia/general/200702/07/P200702070216.htm

Harrington, R., & Pitman, S. (2009). US authorities target phthalates as part of chemical scrutiny overhaul. Retrieved October 9, 2009, from http://www.cosmeticsdesign.com/Formulation-Science/US-authorities-target-phthalates-as-part-of-chemical-scrutiny-overhaul

Hewitt, P.L., & Flett, G.L. (1991). Dimensions of perfectionism in unipolar depression. *Journal of Abnormal Psychology, 100,*98-101.

Hewitt, P.L., & Flett, G.L. (1993). Dimensions of perfectionism, daily stress, and depression: A test of a specific vulnerability hypothesis. *Journal of Abnormal Psychology, 102,*58-65.

Houlihan, J., & Wiles, R. (2000). Beauty Secrets: Does a common chemical in nail polish pose risks to human health? Environmental Working Group.

JiuJik. (2007). Job File 23 Oct 2007. Retrieved October 7, 2009, from http://www.jiujik.com/jsarticle.php?lcid=HK.B5&artid=3000018827&arttype=JOBFI&artsection=CAREER

JUMP. (2009). Career News 20090828. Retrieved October 7, 2009, from http://jump.mingpao.com/cfm/JobArticle1.cfm?PublishDate=2009082 8&TopicID=L9&Filename=gp0900207.txt

Kaschak, E. (1992). Engendered Lives: A New Psychology of Women's Experience. Basic Books.

LeMoncheck, L. (1997). Loose Women, Lecherous Men: A Feminist Philosophy of Sex. Oxford University Press.

McDaniel, S.H. (1988). The interpersonal politics of premenstrual syndrome. *Family Systems Medicine, 6,*134-149.

Parker, K. (2008). 'Save the males': Ho culture lights fuses, but confuses. NY Daily News. Random House.

Pitman, S. (2006a). Cancer lobby group targets nail varnish maker. Retrieved October 9, 2009, http://www.cosmetics design.com/ Formulation-Science/Cancer-lobby-group-targets-nail-varnish-maker

Pitman, S. (2006b). Nail polish manufacturers remove potentially harmful chemicals. Retrieved October 9, 2009, from http://www.cosmetics design.com/Formulation-Science/Nail-Polish-manufacturers-remove-potentially-harmful-chemicals

Pitman, S. (2009). Study suggests risks for beauty care workers exposed to solvents while pregnant. Retrieved October 9, 2009, from http://www. cosmeticsdesign-europe.com/Formulation-Science/Study-suggests-risks-for-beauty-care-workers-exposed-to-solvents-while-pregnant

Saltzberg, E.A., & Chrisler, J.C. (1995). Beauty is the best: Psychological effects of the pursuit of the perfect female body. In J.Freeman (ed.), *Women: A feminist perspective* (5th ed., pp.306-315). Mountain View, CA: Mayfield.

Shroff, H., Reba, L., Thornton, L.M., Tozzi, F., Klump, K.L., & Berrettini, W.H. (2006). Features associated with excessive exercise in women with eating disorders. *International Journal of Eating Disorders, 39,*454-461.

Suarez, S.M., Silvers, D.N., Scher, R.K., Pearlstein, H.H., & Auerbach, R. (1991). Histologic Evaluation of Nail Clippings for Diagnosing Onychomycosis. *Arch Dermatology, 127,*1517-1519.

Ussher, J.M. (2004). Premenstrual syndrome and self-policing: Ruptures in self-silencing lead to increased self-surveillance and blaming of the body. *Social Theory & Health, 2,*254-272.

VTC. (2003). 2003 Manpower Survey Tables Beauty Care, Hairdressing and Cosmetics Industry. Retrieved October 6, 2009, from http://www.vtc.edu.hk/content/68/52/3/Beauty%20table.pdf

VTC. (2009). Prospectus and Admissions 2009. Retrieved October 6, 2009, from http://www.vtc.edu.hk/admission/txt-eng/course/course-06733d.html

Zaias, N. (1990). *The nail in health and disease.* McGraw-Hill.

# Chapter 5

# MICRONEEDLE THERAPY AND HEALTH

## *Zenobia C. Y. Chan and Queeni T. Y. Ip*
The Hong Kong Polytechnic University, China

## ABSTRACT

Undoubtedly the manufacturers of cosmetic products are continuously improving the cutaneous permeation to achieve the prefect facial result. It is believed that higher permeation of hydrophilic active compounds of cosmetic products into the subcutaneous layers of the skin cancels out the dehydrated skin ageing effects. However, the physiological structure of the stratum corneum and the UV exposed lipid-rich cells of facial areas (Wefers et al., 1991) are much less permeable to hydrophilic compound (Birchall, 2006). Moreover lower levels of cutaneous hydration reduce the diffusion of active ingredient into the skin (Doyle et al., 2005). Microneedle therapy or skin needling can remove the lipids from cells and increase the hydrophilic molecule diffusion rate coefficient (Schwindt et al., 1998). Hence the anti-ageing approach can be reached. Certainly there are other benefits resulted from microneedle therapy. But, there are other treatments can achieve certain effects too. It is not the only way for anti ageing. Such self injury facial therapies are sometimes seen as "self-mutilation". There are both supportive and opposite view of "self-mutilation" for this dermabrasion. It is crucial that people without necessary need but seeking this "self-mutilation" should be properly cared. Psychological health risk is hidden under this behavior. Special care and support should be given to the high risk group of beauty therapists or practitioners. Microneedle therapy is now hot in medical beauty industry. And it can be extended to personal use but not professional only. Public can buy the tools on the market easily. Public health education should be addressed and some precautions are discussed for this unmentioned topic.

# INTRODUCTION

Microneedle therapy or skin needling uses a knead rod inlayed with around 200 slender needles, accompanying with functional nutrition liquid, regularly rolling in the places which need to cure, it can puncture more than 250,000 micro vessels on the epidermal within several minutes and form a efficient nutrient delivery system in the epidermis and subcutaneous tissue, with which the active ingredient of the nutrition can entry into skin effectively. Different lengths of needle, usually ranged from 0.1-3.0mm, are chosen for different effects and skin types. Then make skin maintenance, skin care, skin treatment and skin beauty to be perfect. It is one of the hot treatments in medical beauty industry because both the cost and result are effective. It has been used for resurfacing likes stretch marks, injuries ,and acne-scarred and anti-ageing in cosmetic surgeries.

Previously microneedle therapy has long been used by dermatologists in the form of Collagen Induction Therapy (CIT) to fade scars and generally as an anti-ageing treatment. Shortly afterwards smaller sizes of microneedles were recognized for their capacity to dramatically increase the bioavailability of facial treatments and further enhance their transcutaneous absorption.

There are three main advantages of this therapy. First, increasing penetration of actives and facilitating higher serum concentrations at the dermal level. Second, scar reduction, is usually used for acne sufferers as they involve a loss of tissue at the site of the scar, giving the appearances of "holes" in the skin. Third, collagen induction by controlled wounding builds layers of the supporting intracellular matrix which promote healthy, resilient skin that looks younger. The effective beauty result was impressed to beauty industry. It is commonly found for facial treatment on the market.

## LITERATURE REVIEW

Global literatures of dermabrasion is usually about managing depressed scars (Arouete, 1976), quantitative bacterial assessment (Pallua et al., 1999), resurfacing (Fulton & Silverton, 1999), dermatologic surgery (Glazer, 1986), wrinkles (Seltzer, 1976), multiple syringomas (Montalvo et al., 2003), tumescent anesthesia (Breuninger & Wehner-Caroli, 1998), YAG laser (Goldberg, 2000). There is few literature of dermabrasion related to needle (Fabbrocini et al., 2009) and no literature regarding microneedle therapy and health has been published.

One of the most remarkable discoveries for microneedle therapy was probably by a Canadian Plastic Surgeon from scar camouflage tattooing procedures with skin color pigment in patients with hypochromic facial scars. And the appearance of the scars was remarkably improved both in texture and color after one to two years post procedure. Finally, the insertion of the fine tattoo gun needles into the scar managed to break down the scar collagen and lead to a synthesis of new healthy collagen as well as to a re-stimulation of melanogenesis was performed (Camirand & Douchet, 1997).

Although microneedle therapy is hot in medical beauty industry and personally, literature about this area and health lack. These simple tools and easy practice of microneedle therapy are further extended for personal home care use. The dermaroller and facial serum can be easily bought in the market. Although microneedle therapy can be practiced easily, unskillful and improper care would make the negative facial effect. Certain crisis and health problems should be addressed.

Besides microneedle therapy is another "self-injury" behavior follows eyebrow tattooing which internalizes women's psychological health risk. It is argued that female beauty is a self-normalization to feminine culture so as to achieve internal stability. But people without necessary needs and then perform microneedle therapy can be seen as "self mutilation" that is the attention-seeking behavior and escape from intolerable effect (Levenkron, 1998). In extreme, failure and such oppressive societal norms of beauty and femininity are hypothesized as a big bomb that ultimately weakens social mental health. Public health prevention and education must be aware, especially for the high risk beauty therapists or practitioners.


## CONTENT


Beauty science is continuously developed day by day so as to reach the best anti-ageing effect. At the same time, we are ageing second by second. Water, nutrient and other active compounds are running off from inside out and cause different skin problems like wrinkle, dehydrated skin etc. It is believed that beauty products and treatments can compensate the loss from skin. Fundamentally, the basic skin care is putting moisturizing products onto the skin. Active ingredients of products will be released and permeate from the epidermal skin into the subcutaneous layers of the skin (Higuchi, 1960) through the three natural transdermal delivery routes, that is the stratum corneum, hair follicle pores and sebaceous gland canals to achieve rejuvenation theoretically. However, the watery products are limited by the physical diffusion (Smith, 2004). The physiological structure of the stratum corneum (Wille, 2006) and the UV exposed lipid-rich cells of facial areas (Wefers et al., 1991) are much less permeable to hydrophilic compound (Birchall, 2006). Moreover lower levels of cutaneous hydration reduce the diffusion of active ingredient into the skin (Doyle et al., 2005). Hence the permeation is barricaded. Microneedle therapy can remove the lipids from cells and increase the hydrophilic molecule diffusion rate coefficient (Schwindt et al., 1998). There are evidences that microneedle therapy can improve the cutaneous permeation (Ferguson & O'Kane, 2004; Oh et al., 2008; Verbaan et al., 2007).

Apart from the penetration enhancement, scar reduction can be done by microneedle therapy as well. Scar tissue is formed when damaged layers of epidermis are repaired rapidly in the presence of TGF-$\beta$1 & 2. It is showed that scar can be inhibited if TGF-$\beta$1 & 2 decreases (Ferguson, & O'Kane, 2004). Also, scar can be found more often in old people as the level of TGF-$\beta$1 & 2 increases in mature skin. Therefore, a different healing can be resulted by microneedling as small injuries and inhibition of TGF-$\beta$1 & 2 can be controlled and therefore scar formation would not caused.

Moreover, microneedle treatments have been shown to induce collagen formation (Wu et al., 2008) but not hyperpigmentation as they do not remove the epidermis (Cho et al., 2008). Therefore microneedle therapy promotes healing with less damage and recovery time than traditional ablative or other re-surfacing techniques (Aust et al., 2008 b). It used to fade the flaws. When the wounds from the surgery are closed the microneedle roller can be used safely and will encourage faster healing with less scarring and no significant adverse effects were noted in any patient (Majid, 2009).

Collagen synthesis is complex and occurs in different ways in different areas of the body (Fernandes & Signorini, 2008; Hulmes, 1992; 2002), but epidermal collagen can be stimulated by injury. Collagen Induction Therapy is based on the skin's inherent repair response to mechanical injury that the damaged collagen and elastin are recycled to produce more regular layers of tissue and new collagen is synthesized immediately (Aust et al., 2008 a). Microneedle therapy allows for the controlled induction of the skin's self repair mechanism, by creating micro injuries in the skin, which induce new collagen synthesis to a controlled degree (Aust et al., 2008 a & b).

All the above advantages make microneedle therapy popular in the medical beauty industry. And the cost and result effective way initiate another hot trend to Hong Kong beauty industry after the lasing or radio frequent treatment. A microneedle therapy can be performed with approximate several hundreds to thousand Hong Kong dollars in the beauty market. This price is not much different to the common facial treatment. The low entry fee but great "return" of that "special" treatment is quite welcome to the clients although there are higher risks compare to the basic facial treatments. In addition, simply tools and uses cause further extension to personal home care use. Hundreds to thousands dollars for the cost of the microneedle therapy kit set is even attractive to them. Nevertheless, contraindications, precautions and risks are hidden. It is accepted that people pursue different beauty treatments based on the perfectionism and self-normalization theories which have been discussed in the previous chapters. The main reason and force behind for different beauty treatments is the beautification. It is also understood why people suffer different skin problems did the microneedle therapy. However, there are other similar effects and safe beauty treatments rather than microneedling in the market. It is curious that people would like to beautify themselves only without other necessary needs are still seeking this high risk "self-injury" treatment. It is dangerous that psychological health risk behind such behavior.

## DISCUSSION

Although there are many advantages of microneedle therapy, the risk is still comparative higher than other beauty treatments with similar effect. It is understood that people with necessary needs like acne sufferers would seek this high risk therapy for better beautification. However, it is curious that people without necessary needs are still seeking this high risk therapy rather than other safer beauty treatments. It is not the only way to get the good result. Microneedle therapy is done by self injury process which is a self harm or mutilation behavior.

Favazza and Rosenthal (1993) identify pathological self-mutilation as the deliberate alteration or destruction of body tissue without conscious suicidal intent. The person who self-harms often has difficulty experiencing feelings of anxiety, anger, or sadness. Consequently cutting or disfiguring the skin serves as a coping mechanism. The injury is intended to assist the individual in dissociating from immediate tension (Stanley et al., 2001).

Microneedle therapy seems to be "self-mutilation". But Levenkron (1998) argues that behavior is not typical of self-mutilation. The majority of these persons tolerate pain for the purpose of attaining a finished product like a piercing or tattoo. This differs from the individual who self-mutilates for whom pain experienced from cutting or damaging skin is sought as an escape from intolerable effect.

From my point of view, people bear "normal" skin and without necessary needs but they are still seeking such "self-harm" microneedle therapy can be counted as self mutilation. In the result oriented and time efficient Hong Kong society, beauty effect is the most dominate among other considerations It is observed that they are escaping the ageing effect, they are anxious about old. Keeping young is important and evens everything in their lives. To escape the depression from ageing problems including wrinkles, dry and dull skin, etc., they will to try the vigorous and high risk microneedle therapy and forget other gentle ways. Focusing and repeating microneedle therapy further induce cosmetic addiction. Health prevention and education should emphasis the concept and attitude of facing ageing. It is also observed that the high risk group of self mutilating beauty treatment may be the beauty therapists or practitioners because they are mostly pay more attention and put more weight on their appearances. As they are the pioneers to get touch with these new technologies, they usually try first without in-depth study and enough precautions. Their working objectives are concentrating on anti-ageing. It is worry about that they will be psychological illness. It is understood that active facing ageing psychologically is difficultly be promoted and educated in the beauty industry which focus on anti-ageing all the way. But they must be first targeted and educated, else they cannot bring the message of physical and psychological health to their clients correctly and public health is further affected. In extreme, beauty industry may be deteriorated and shrunk finally.

Nevertheless, public are still "enjoying" the pain therapy and the use has been extended to home care. Public can easily buy the dermaroller and concentrated serum for self use without any prescriptions. It is dangerous that public may not choose the suitable roller and right solution for themselves. Dermaroller has a variety of needle length for optimum results. They may not handle the dermaroller well and cause harms. Longer needles can cause more damage and longer healing time but deeper tissue can be stimulated. It is dangerous that longer needles were used on the sensitive, thin and delicate skin. Longer needles are used by professional while short needles are recommended for beginner.

Apart from the needle length, the material of the needle is another important topic. Titanium gives a finer edge that lasts much longer and preventing excess irritation caused by blunted needles is much better than the stainless steel. The titanium needles are also gold-plated to help inhibit microbial growth and maintain sterility. The gold coating also prevents oxidation and pitting of the surface even with long term use. This is especially important for non-single-use products that penetrate the skin's surface. A sanitizing solution is also available and is recommended for sanitizing rollers pre-use. Moreover, the serum after open should be handled well to prevent contamination or denaturation.

More pressure for the microneedles to enter the skin causes more pain for the same penetration depth. Before skillful practice, inaccurate pressure may be forced to make unnecessary pain and harm. UV explosion especially suntan and all irritable facial action must be stopped in that period. Special care and products should be used after microneedle therapy. Otherwise, injure and harm may be caused.


## CONCLUSION

Although there are many advantages of microneedle therapy including cutaneous permeation enhancement, scar reduction, collagen induction, effective cost and result etc., the risk is comparative higher than other beauty treatments with similar effect. Microneedle therapy is not the only way to improve the skin quality. It is wonder why people who will to suffer unnecessary pain from microneedle therapy but not the other comfortable and effective facial treatments. It should not be counted with both effective result and cost only. People without necessary needs but still bear the pain experience and infectious risk for seeking better skin should be aware. Psychological illness and cosmetic addiction may be initiated by such "self mutilation" to escape the ageing anxiety and achieve internal balance Microneedle therapy is now popular in beauty industry and has been self-used commonly. Some precautions have been discussed. Public health education and prevention of facing ageing attitude should be promoted especially to the beauty front liners though it contrasts to the anti-ageing concept of beauty industry. Hope other health educators and promoters can put more weight and resources on the beauty sector so that beauty and health can be grown in directly proportion to aim the real beauty and health industry ultimately.

# REFERENCES

Arouete, J. (1976). Correction of depressed scars on the face by a method of elevation. *J Dermatol Surg, 2*(4),337-339.

Aust, M.C., Fernandes, D., Kolokythas, P., Kaplan, H.M., & Vogt, P.M. (2008 a). Percutaneous Collagen Induction Therapy: An Alternative Treatment for Scars, Wrinkles, and Skin Laxity. *Plastic and Reconstructive Surgery, 121*(4),1421-1429.

Aust, M.C., Reimers, K., Repenning, C., Stahl, F., Jahn, S., Guggenheim, M., Schwaiger, N., Gohritz, A., & Vogt, P.M. (2008 b). Percutaneous collagen induction: minimally invasive skin rejuvenation without risk of hyperpigmentation - fact or fiction? *Plastic and Reconstructive Surgery, 122*(5),1553-1563.

Birchall, J.C. (2006). Stratum Corneum Bypassed or Removed. *Enhancement in Drug Delivery*, 337.

Breuninger, H., & Wehner-Caroli, J. (1998). Slow infusion tumescent anesthesia. *Dermatol Surg, 24*(7),759-763.

Camirand, A., & Douchet, J. (1997). Needle Dermabrasion. *Aesthetic Plast Surg, 21*,48-51.

Cho, S.B., Lee, S.J., Kang, J.M., Kim, Y.K., Kim, T.Y., & Kim, D.H. (2008). The treatment of burn scar-induced contracture with the pinhole method and collagen induction therapy: a case report. *Journal of the European Academy of Dermatology & Venereology, 22*(4),513.

Doyle, D., Hanks, G.., Cherny, N.I., & Calman, K. (2005). *7 Principles of drug delivery in Pallative Medicine. Oxford textbook of palliative medicine* (3rd ed.). Oxford University Press.

Fabbrocini, G., Fardella, N., Monfrecola, A., Proietti, I., & Innocenzi, D. (2009). Acne scarring treatment using skin needling. *Clinical and Experimental Dermatology, 34*(8),874-879.

Favazza, A.R., & Rosenthal, R.J. (1993). Diagnostic issues in self-mutilation. *Hospital & Community Psychiatry, 44*,134-140.

Ferguson, M.W.J., & O'Kane, S. (2004). *Scar-free healing: from embryonic mechanisms to adult therapeutic intervention.* Philosophical Transactions of the Royal Society of London. Series B: Biological Sciences. *359*(1445),839-850.

Fernandes, D., & Signorini, M. (2008). Combating photoaging with percutaneous collagen induction. *Clinics in Dermatology, 26*(2),192-199.

Fulton, J.E., & Silverton, K. (1999). Resurfacing the acne-scarred face. *Dermatol Surg, 25*(5),353-359.

Glazer, S.F. (1986). An overview of dermatologic surgery. *Compr Ther, 12*(5),32-37.

Goldberg, D.J. (2000). Full-face nonablative dermal remodeling with a 1320 nm Nd:YAG laser. *Dermatol Surg, 26*(10),915-918.

Higuchi, T. (1960). Physical chemical analysis of precutaneous absorption process from creams and ointments. *J Soc Cosmet Chem, 11*,85-97.

Hulmes, D.J. (2002). Building collagen molecules, fibrils, and suprafibrillar structures. *Journal of Structural Biology, 137*(1-2),2-10.

Hulmes, D.J. (1992). The collagen superfamily—diverse structures and assemblies. *Essays in Biochemistry, 27*,49-67.

Levenkron, S. (1998). *Cutting.* New York, NY: W. W. Norton and Company.

Majid, I. (2009). *Microneedling therapy in atrophic facial scars: An objective assessment.* Cutis Skin and Laser Clinic, Govt Medical College, Srinagar, India. *2*(1),26-30.

Montalvo, K., Matthews, J., & Graham, B. (2003). Multiple syringomas in an unusual distribution. *Skinmed, 2*(5),322-323.

Oh, J.H., Park, H.H., Doa, K.Y., Han, M., Hyun, D.H., Kim, C.G., Kim, C.H., Lee, S.S., Hwang, S.J., Shin, S.C., & Cho, C.W. (2008). Influence of the delivery systems using a microneedle array on the permeation of a hydrophilic molecule, calcein. *European Journal of Pharmaceutics and Biopharmaceutics, 69*(3),1040-1045.

Pallua, N., Fuchs, P.C., Hafemann, B., Völpel, U., Noah, M., & Lütticken, R. (1999). A new technique for quantitative bacterial assessment on burn wounds by modified dermabrasion. *J Hosp Infect, 42*(4),329-337.

Schwindt, D.A., Wilhelm, K.P., & Maibach, H.I. (1998). Water diffusion characteristics of human stratum corneum at different anatomical sites in vivo. *Journal of Investigative Dermatology, 111*(3),385-389.

Smith, W.F. (2004). *Foundations of Materials Science and Engineering* (3rd ed.). McGraw-Hill.

Stanley, B., Gameroff, M.J., Michaelson, V., & Mann, J.J. (2001). Are suicide attempters who self-mutilate a unique population? *American Journal of Psychiatry, 158*(3),427-432.

Seltzer, A.P. (1976). Wrinkles around the mouth: needle treatment. *J Natl Med Assoc, 68*(4),323-324.

Verbaan, F.J., Bal, S.M., van den Berg, D.J., Groenink, W.H.H., Verpoorten, H., Lüttge, R., & Bouwstra, J.A. (2007). Assembled microneedle arrays enhance the transport of compounds varying over a large range of molecular weight across human dermatomed skin. *Journal of Controlled Release, 117*(2),238-245.

Wefers, H., Melnik, B.C., Flür, M., Bluhm, C., Lehmann, P., & Plewig, G. (1991). Influence of UV irradiation on the composition of human stratum corneum lipids. *Journal of Investigative Dermatology*, *96*(6),959-962.

Wille, J.J. (2006). *Skin Delivery Systems: Transermals, Dermatologicals, and Cosmetic Actives* (1st ed.). Blackwell Publishing.

Wu, Y., Qiu, Y., & Zhang, S. (2008). Microneedle-based drug delivery: studies on delivery parameters and biocompatibility. *Biomedical Microdevices*, *10*(5),601-610.

# Chapter 6

# STEM-CELL COSMETICS

## *Zenobia C. Y. Chan and Queeni T. Y. Ip*

The Hong Kong Polytechnic University, China

## ABSTRACT

Traditionally, healthcare services and aesthetics have been treated as two separate industries. Nowadays, however, beauty is interpreted as implying health (Alam & Dover, 2001). Beauties must be relatively healthy because beauty is a physiological burden that only a strong body can support (Hamilton & Zuk, 1982). Nancy Etcoff argued that beauty is a universal part of human experience that helps ensure the survival of our genes (Etcoff, 1999). Genetic aesthetic modification is being developed. Use of stem-cell technology is now hot in the beauty industry, involving stimulating the proliferation of stem-cells to continuously repair and replenish damaged epidermal skin cells. Indeed, true beauty may not be promoted from the inside out to restore health and wellness. There are no literature regarding stem-cell cosmetics and health has been published in Hong Kong. Many unexplored rooms and hidden risks of this therapy should be studied. Although stem-cell cosmetics therapy can raise the quality of life in the coming dominated elderly population, health prevention, and education should promote the unbiased appraisal of stem-cell cosmetics at the same time for public before taking action.

## INTRODUCTION

Inevitable ageing happens in all the life of the world. Age, this word involves different complicated meanings. Meaning old and implying devaluation which link health and beauty together. Negative meanings about declining activity, poor health status, deteriorating physical appearance, outdated mind, lower working efficiency, limited time and life span, etc. cause anti-aging finally comes out and be emphasized in both health and beauty industries in order to achieve positive competiveness in the modern society especially in Hong Kong where is always pursuing fast and efficiency.

Directly control of the body to the removal of the signs of ageing. To control fundamental intra-cellular processes where the objective is to extend or break the limits to the human life span (Vincent, 2007). Stem-cell technology was used.

Stem-cells are a type of cell which has the unique ability to develop into various types of tissue like muscle, skin, nerve, brain, etc. There are also a variety of other stem-cell sources which do not involve the use of human embryos. It is common that stem-cell can be obtained from liposuction. The regenerative cells can then be used to repair the damaged cells. The concept of stem-cell technology was applied in cosmetic way. It is believed in the efficacy of adult stem-cell therapies and plans on initially focusing its efforts in the beauty market providing minimally invasive treatments which are intended to be a natural and lower-risk alternative to many current therapies or as additional treatments to existing ones.

The trend of stem-cell cosmetic therapy has been started in the Hong Kong beauty industry following that of microneedle therapy. This relative new technology started several years ago. Stem-cell beauty treatment usually involves a plant extracted stem-cells serum that penetrates into facial skin via an ultra sound device. Now, however, stem-cell injection is going to replace the traditional method, executed by beauty therapists only and commonly found in the beauty salon. Stem-cells are extracted from the client or other sources and injected back into the skin after processing. The price ranges from several hundred to thousands of dollars. Silicone implantation can also be replaced by growing new tissue through the use of stem-cells in cosmetic surgery to decrease the body rejection.

Stem-cell therapy is one of the medical beauty treatments that is equal to medication. The explosion of different unmonitored stem-cell products on the market will cause another wave of medical beauty accidents like those that have resulted from laser therapy and cosmetic surgery. A flood of complaints will be the result (Consumer Council, 2001).

Although the stem-cell cosmetics therapy can relieve the ageing problems, it is foreseeable to result beauty accident, complaint and other coming psychological ill health from this biotechnological beauty therapy if shadow understanding. Anti-ageing cannot be achieved in a holistic way only by the stem-cell technology. Healthy life is also important for anti-age. There is no literature about stem-cell cosmetics therapy and health. And many other countries are also facing the problems from the ageing population in the world. This chapter aims to bring out the information and precautions of stem-cell cosmetics therapy, predict the trend of Hong Kong beauty industry in the coming future, emphasis anti-ageing attitude and importance of real beauty and health through the trendy cosmetic therapy.

## LITERATURE REVIEW

Global stem-cell researches are usually about plastic surgery (Yoshimura et al., 2008), characterization, and isolation (Gimble & Guilak, 2003; Gudjonsson et al., 2002; Ohyama et al., 2006), bone marrow (Kern et al, 2006), differentiation (Daisuke et al., 2005), yield, and growth characteristics of adipose tissue-derived mesenchymal stem-cells (Oedayrajsingh-Varma et al., 2006), alternative stem-cell source (Hattoria et al., 2004), stem-cell factor (De Paulis et al., 1999). There are few literatures about stem-cell and cosmetic use.

Adipose-derived stem-cells (ADSCs) and their secretory factors can stimulate collagen synthesis and migration of fibroblasts during the wound healing process. Conventional treatments for skin aging, such as lasers and topical regimens, induce new collagen synthesis via activation of dermal fibroblasts or growth factors (Fraser et al., 2006). It is studied that ADSCs can also be used for the treatment of skin aging. ADSCs produce many useful growth factors, increase collagen production in animal study, and reverse skin aging in human trial. ADSCs and their secretory factors show promise for application in cosmetic dermatology, especially in the treatment of skin aging (Park et al, 2008).

Research has also shown that inserting a gene for the protein component of telomerase into senescent human cells re-extends their telomeres to lengths typical of young cells, and the cells then display all the other identifiable characteristics of young and healthy cells. This advance not only suggests that telomeres are the central timing mechanism for cellular aging, but also demonstrates that such a mechanism can be reset, extending the replicative life span of such cells and resulting in markers of gene expression typical of "younger", i.e. early passage, cells without the hallmarks of malignant transformation. It is now possible to explore the fundamental cellular mechanisms underlying human aging, clarifying the role played by replicative senescence (Fossel, 1998).

Nevertheless, research about stem-cell cosmetics therapy and anti-ageing is still in its early stages, and clinical trials on humans are rare (Parfitt, 2005). Stem-cell cosmetics and health is seldom discussed. It is very serious to emphasis its importance that unlike other non-invasive beauty treatment. Invasive stem-cell cosmetics can cause huge harms and impact to the public health as it involves the biotechnological level. Careless action of that invasive beauty treatment may cause illness likes cancer (Parfitt, 2005). In addition, stem-cell beauty and health is close relationship. It is undoubtedly that stem-cell technology can give advantages on the coming elderly population in the world. A public health challenge to provide increased quality of life for this growing segment of the population requires more attention to the variable of age in experimental studies. Stem-cell populations are likely to be a fruitful subject (Van Zantab & Liang, 2003). More public health prevention and education should be promoted regarding the stem-cell beauty as well in order to raise the living standard.

# CONTENT

Stem-cell technology has been applied in cosmetic surgery industry earlier than beauty industry. Regenerative cells are obtained through the remarkable potential of the fat tissue in our bodies. Although the technique of fat grafting in plastic surgery has been around for years, the capability of our body's regenerative cells to provide a more natural and consistent result is a recent breakthrough in cosmetic enhancement. Regenerative cell fat transfer is taking high-demand cosmetic procedures to the next level. Regenerative cell enhanced fat grafting simply transfers excess soft fat tissue from one part of the body to the part where enhancement is desired. Fat tissue is obtained through a standard liposuction procedure and is then processed through cutting-edge technology to separate out regenerative cells. Regenerative cells are then ready to be reinserted into the desired area of the body.

The regenerative cell technique and fat grafting promotes tissue survival, graft retention, and increased volume, making it more effective than traditional procedures. The use of the regenerative cells in the graft enables the transplanted fat to successfully integrate with the surrounding tissue much better than with previous methods. There is no risk of rejection by the body, because the procedure uses your own tissue and cells. There are many areas of body like face, chin, breast, skin, and scars that can benefit significantly from regenerative cell enhanced fat grafting.

The use of stem-cell cosmetics therapy is then being extended in the beauty industry. Although the autologus cell regeneration, i.e. own-cell, is not very common, the acceptance of this therapy is broadening. On the other hand, different products and ways of stem-cell cosmetics therapy have been applied. It is commonly that stem-cell from plant has been extracted and processed to produce as a bottle of concentrated serum which then be used with ultrasound device or microneedle therapy for dermal penetration. Besides, stem-cell elements have been added into different skin care and home care products to enhance their effects.

At the same time, autologous stem-cell banking, the use of your own cells for treatment, is the only way to ensure that there is a genetic stem-cell match when stem-cells are needed for a medical procedure. Often, patients are recommended by their physicians for a stem-cell transplant as an only option to treating their illness without waiting a very long time from an appropriate donor who may be someone with a close genetic match. Even in instances where a donor can be found, patient conditions may worsen drastically and, in many cases, some individuals may never find a match, therefore making the therapy impossible. This experience may be avoided by having your own banked stem-cells before the onset of disease. Autologous stem-cell transplants also eliminate the need for immunosuppressant therapy which is required when a donor is involved. Patients succumb to a lifetime of prescription drugs in order to ward off their own body rejecting the cell transplant. When autologous cells are transplanted, no medications of this kind are generally needed.

The same concept has also been applied in medical beauty industry. Pre-disease collection, processing and long-term storage of adult stem-cells for the general population has been started to use for future beauty applications or repair the damaged or aged cell. Anti-ageing skin care problems can be relieved. Generating revenue through ongoing fees associated with a minimally invasive, proprietary stem-cell collection process, in addition to fees charged to the centers for marketing and long-term storage. Beauty and health conscious consumers have been targeted to encourage them to donate and store their stem-cells as a form of bio-insurance for possible use in later years or to address an emerging medical and beauty need. Stem-cell banking services have been made affordable through a financing program which allows clients to participate in a monthly payment plan without interest. The monthly fee includes the collection, processing, cryopreservation (freezing), and storage. Other plans are also available to extend the months of payment and lower the monthly fees.

Such marketing strategies promote stem-cell cosmetics therapy will be dominated in the medical beauty market. Such research and development will be continuously improved. It is foreseeable that autologus skin care products will be tailor made for client in the coming future.

## DISCUSSION

Hong Kong people pursue fast and efficiency. Cosmetic powders and traditional facial treatment seem to be faded out through competition in the development of Hong Kong beauty industry. Medical beauty is now dominated with the evidence of different medical facial treatments like lasing and microneedle therapy.

It is no doubt that anti-age can be benefited from the stem-cell cosmetic therapy. Its precautions should also be aware. Stem-cell concentrate or product has been mostly packaged into natural product because the stem-cell has been extracted from plants, from natural. It is even promoted to zero harm beauty product. The use as a medical plant and its advantage are emphasized. Natural is not equal to no harm. In fact, it is the product of biochemistry. It is worried that public may be side tracked and do not understand of real stem-cell cosmetics deeply. Product label is recommended for such stem-cell product to public. Besides, the concentrate has been claimed to be ionized. Its stability and activity are questioned. They may not give the effect as they claimed.

Besides the ingredients and effect of plant extracted stem-cell products, it is worried about where the stem-cell extracts go after injection. The extracts may not "arrive" the treated area. No one knows the outcome of stem-cell therapy in different clients, the sources of stem-cells, the hygiene and safety of the process, its relationship with carcinoma and other infections, or what the side effects are. The professor running the state-authorized adult stem-cell bank is concerned that patients are effectively paying to be guinea pigs for untested treatments. One major concern is that patients are being injected with a blend of tissues from aborted foetuses or other material of questionable origin (Parfitt, 2005). It is also wondered if the ability of stem-cell is still work or functional after storage. All may be hazardous to the public health, which is totally unprotected.

Moreover, ethical and moral controversy, reputation of manufacturer, product labeling, legal and right, further legislation and monitor, and insurance have not been directly instructed in details. And all these issues about stem-cell cosmetics therapy are different in different countries. Attention should be paid on.

Stem-cell cosmetics therapy is trendy after microneedle therapy in beauty industry. It is believed that stem-cell technology will be continuously researched and developed. Science and technology is laddered and applied in the beauty industry. It is possible that people whose explicit aim to achieve immortality and forever beauty exist, no longer rejuvenation only in the coming future. Commercial products and technical devices offer to keep your body frozen until science has progressed sufficiently to revive you and keep you alive (Shostak, 2002). Senescence may become the history in the end of beauty science ultimately.

Before the above revolutionary success, as life expectancy in industrialized countries increases, appropriate care of elderly skin looms as a dermatologic priority. Skin ageing is a complex, multifactorial process whose baseline rate is genetically determined but that may be accelerated by environmental, mechanical, or socioeconomic factors. The intrinsic structural changes that occur with the aging of the skin increase skin fragility, decrease the ability of the skin to heal, increase risk for toxicological injuries, promote the development of various cutaneous disorders, and produce aesthetically undesirable effects like wrinkling and uneven pigmentation. As aged patients represent a larger segment of the population, increased attention to the problems of the aged skin, both cosmetic and beyond, will be necessary and should build on currently successful interventions to improve their quality of life (Farage et al., 2007).

# CONCLUSION

The use of cosmetics, cosmetic surgery, hair dyes, and similar means for covering up in today's society in order to increase the competitiveness. Genetic engineering, stem-cells, geriatric medicine, and therapeutic pharmaceuticals have been researched enthusiastically to produce an anti-aging medicine (Olshansky et al., 2002). Stem-cells cosmetics therapy and product have also been inspired in the beauty industry. And its need is foreseen to increase with the elderly population. In fact, ageing is complex. It is caused by many factors like stress, diet, environment etc.. It is no doubt that stem-cell cosmetic therapy is a way to rejuvenate. But the most important of maintain anti-ageing should be prevention to maintain good health and young holistically. Regular diet and exercise should not be ignored. Behavioral change is important for prevention. It is hoped that the aim of beauty and health would not be side tracked by the anti-ageing medical beauty treatment. Therefore, public health prevention and promotion should be enhanced to show the importance and correlation of beauty and health. Research about stem-cell cosmetics therapy and anti-ageing is still in its early stages, and clinical trials on humans are rare (Parfitt, 2005). Efforts to prevent accidents resulting from beauty therapies should never cease. We foresee a chain of cause and effect that will bring repeated problems to the medical healthcare sector. Stem-cell cosmetics therapy is marketing and selling in prevention which is also imported in public health education and promotion. Public health education and prevention should promote the precautions and risk so that the quality of life will not be obstructed by the expected therapy.

# REFERENCES

Alam, M., & Dover, J.S. (2001). On Beauty: Evolution, Psychosocial Considerations, and Surgical Enhancement. *Arch Dermatol, 137,*795-807.

Daisuke, S., Joji, M., Toru, I., Takuya, W., Tomoko, N., Kiyoshi, A., & Tomomitsu, H. (2005). Differentiation of Mesenchymal Stem-cells Transplanted to a Rabbit Degenerative Disc Model: Potential and Limitations for Stem-cell Therapy in Disc Regeneration. *Spine*, *30*(21),2379-2387.

De Paulis, A., Minopoli, G., Arbustini, E., de Crescenzo, G., Piaz, F.D., Pucci, P., Russo, T., & Marone, G. (1999). Stem-cell Factor Is Localized in, Released from, and Cleaved by Human Mast Cells. *The Journal of Immunology*, *163*, 2799-2808.

Etcoff, N. (1999). Survival of the Prettiest: The Science of Beauty. New York, NY: Doubleday.

Farage, M.A., Miller, K.W., Elsner, P., & Maibach, H.I. (2007). Structural Characteristics of the Aging Skin: A Review. *Cutaneous and Ocular Toxicology*, *26*(4), 343-357.

Fraser, J.K., Wulur, I., Alfonso, Z., & Hedrick, M.H. (2006). Fat tissue: an underappreciated source of stem-cells for biotechnology. *TRENDS in Biotechnology*, *24*(4),150-154.

Fossel, M. (1998). Telomerase and the Aging Cell. Implications for Human Health. *JAMA*, *279*,1732-1735.

Gimble, J.M., & Guilak, F. (2003). Adipose-derived adult stem-cells: isolation, characterization, and differentiation potential. *Cytotherapy*, *5*(5),362-369.

Gudjonsson, T., Villadsen, R., Nielsen, H.L., Rønnov-Jessen, L., Bissell, M.J., & Petersen, O.W. (2002). Isolation, immortalization, and characterization of a human breast epithelial cell line with stem-cell properties. *Genes & Dev, 16*,693-706.

Hamilton, W.D., & Zuk, M. (1982). Heritable true fitness and bright birds: a role for parasites? *Science*, *218*,384-387.

Hattoria, H., Satod, M., Masuokab, K., Ishiharac, M., Kikuchib, T., Matsuia, T., Takasea, B., Ishizukaa, T., Kikuchic, M., Fujikawab, K., & Ishihara, M. (2004). Osteogenic Potential of Human Adipose Tissue-Derived Stromal Cells as an Alternative Stem-cell Source. *Cells Tissues Organs*, *178*,2-12.

Kern, S., Eichler, H., Stoeve, J., Klüter, H., & Bieback, K. (2006). Comparative Analysis of Mesenchymal Stem-cells from Bone Marrow, Umbilical Cord Blood, or Adipose Tissue. *Stem-cells, 24*(5), 1294-1301.

Oedayrajsingh-Varma, M., van Ham, S., Knippenberg, M., Helder, M., Klein-Nulend, J., Schouten, T., Ritt, M., & van Milligen, F. (2006). Adipose tissue-derived mesenchymal stem-cell yield and growth characteristics are affected by the tissue-harvesting procedure. *Cytotherapy, 8*(2),166-177.

Ohyama, M., Terunuma, A., Tock, C.L., Radonovich, M.F., Pise-Masison, C.A., Hopping, S.B., Brady, J.N., Udey, M.C., & Vogel, J.C. (2006). Characterization and isolation of stem-cell–enriched human hair follicle bulge cells. *Clin Invest, 116*(1),249-260.

Olshansky, S.J., Hayflick, L., & Carnes, B.A. (2002). Position Statement on Human Aging. *Aging Knowl. Environ, 2002*(24),9.

Parfitt, T. (2005). Russian scientists voice concern over "stem-cell cosmetics". *Lancet, 365*,1219-1220.

Park, B.S., Jang, K.A., Sung, J.H., Park, J.S., Kwon, Y.H., Kim, K.J., & Kim, W.S. (2008). Adipose-Derived Stem-cells and Their Secretory Factors as a Promising Therapy for Skin Aging. *Dermatol Surg, 34*,1323-1326.

Shostak, S. (2002) *Becoming Immortal: Combining Cloning and Stem-cell Therapy*. Albany: State University of New York Press.

Storage & Therapies for Umbilical Cord Blood & Stem-cell: Efficacy and Effectiveness in Question - CHOICE # 406. 2001. Consumer Council. Web site: http://www.consumer. org.hk/website/ws_en/ news/press eleases/p40602.html

Van Zantab, G., & Liang, Y. (2003). The role of stem-cells in aging. *Experimental Hematology, 31*(8),659-672.

Vincent, J.A. (2007). Science and imagery in the 'war on old age'. Ageing and Society. Cambridge University Press.

Yoshimura, K., Sato, K., Aoi, N., Kurita, M., Hirohi, T., & Harii, K. (2008). Cell-Assisted Lipotransfer for Cosmetic Breast Augmentation: Supportive Use of Adipose-Derived Stem/Stromal Cells. *Aesthetic Plastic Surgery, 32*(1),48-55.

# Chapter 7

# ANTI-AGEING: HEALTH AND BEAUTY ISSUE

## *Zenobia C. Y. Chan and Queeni T. Y. Ip*
The Hong Kong Polytechnic University, China

## ABSTRACT

Aging is inevitable. Anti-ageing must go on tackling it. Youth and beauty is understandably to preserve but no longer wrinkle elimination only. Anti-ageing should be a preventative health care topic in the coming future because of the growing elderly population. International different professionals from around world, including scientists, physicians, gerontologists, health care practitioners, medical center directors, spa and clinic owners, and those interested and knowledgeable in the field of anti-ageing should be involved to overcome the age related problems. There is no literature of anti-ageing has been published in Hong Kong. Anti ageing has just begun in Hong Kong. Other related health preventative interventions should be co-organized to give more suitable and updated information and support to different age groups which have different needs and preventions for ageing. Earlier plan for suitable public anti ageing can enhance the long term social development and decrease the social expenses and burden.

# INTRODUCTION

Biological progression cannot be stopped before the science of biological immortality (Shostak, 2002) would be maturely developed. A youth appearance is perceived to preserve for more social activities. Youthfulness provides an edge in the capitalist workplace and appearance dependence is nearly inevitable. Dependence on a youthful appearance when such an appearance is waning creates conflict within the individual and dissatisfaction results. This dissatisfaction leads to consumption and furthers interests external to the individual (Bayer, 2004). Anti-ageing science and technology applied by beauty industry offers advancement for public in age resistance. Images in the media foster an aesthetic ideology of the masses that drives the consumption of anti-aging products and services. With the growing elderly population in Hong Kong, anti-ageing is correlated with the social economy and long term development while it is highly correlated with health as well. Anti-age is no longer about wrinkle elimination only. It is no doubt that public anti-ageing work is not prevented by beauty industry only. Physicians from every medical discipline, scientists, nutritionists, gerontologists, chiropractors, pharmacists, pharmaceutical chemists and research, specialists, RNs or nurse practitioners, naturopathic doctors, dentists, bariaticians or weight management specialists, and complementary practitioners of all disciplines should be included. This chapter aims to bring out the message that anti-ageing is one of the big topics of health prevention and promotion. It will impact the social economy and long term development. It is important that anti-age should be lead by preventative health care section. Co-operation of different primary health care and beauty practitioners should be the predicted result. Earlier plan to stay young should be educated to public and supported by government so that high quality of elder living standard and good social development would be enhanced.

## Literature Review

Multiple studies link personal appearance to positive reactions from others including friendship preference, romantic attraction, promotion and success in business (Buss & Schmitt, 1993; Collins & Zebrowitz, 1995). Beauty enhancement is demanded to experience. But there is no literature discussed anti-ageing and health prevention. Global literatures of anti-age are usually about advertisements (Calasanti, 2007), medicinal plants (Hoareau & DaSilva, 1999; Joshi, 2006), anti-ageing factors (Bayer, 2004), marketing (Haberer, 2010). In fact, anti-age is not only talking about physically deterioration, beauty products, anti wrinkle treatments and cosmetic surgery. This topic can extend to psychological health, public health and even social health.

Age affects psychological health is involved. In an online poll, Popular Demographics asked adults to rank their level of happiness with their personal appearance, and on a scale of 1 to 10 (with 1 being least happy), nearly half of the 2510 respondents (47 percent) gave themselves a score of 5 or lower. The poll found that 87 percent of adults say that if they could change any part of their body for cosmetic reasons, they would; half would change multiple body parts. Only few are happy enough with their bodies that they would not change a thing (Fetio, 2003). Statistics suggest that adults, particularly boomers, are dissatisfied and spending their income to make age-defying, cosmetic alterations in unprecedented numbers.

Public health and social health can be further impacted as there is a relationship between youth and vitality. Young people have energy, and energy level reduces with age. In a capitalist society such as America, where an individual's worth is often measured by his/her capacity to produce, energy is highly valued. Not only do the young have more years ahead of them to work, but it is assumed that they are more productive during actual working hours. In producing themselves as workers, individuals become commodities, and a youthful appearance can increase their exchange value in the job market (Bayer, 2004).

CBSnews (2003) states that many boomers are surrounded by younger colleagues or find themselves dating again, they want every part of their bodies to project an image of vitality.

There are lots of literatures about ageing but not anti-ageing. Anti-ageing is not strange but it is still green in concern. Anti-ageing is very important with health in the long term development with the growing population of elders. There is no literature about anti ageing beauty and health care has been published in Hong Kong. Hope this pioneer article of anti-ageing can give insight to the related researchers and preventative health education and promotion for further studies.

## CONTENT

### Aging and Health

Foucault (1973) said the aged body became reduced to a state of degeneration where the meanings of old age and the body's deterioration seemed condemned to signify each other in perpetuity. By recreating death as a phenomenon in life, rather than of life, medical research on aging became separate from the earlier treatises that focused on the promise of longevity. While Katz (1996) lists three commanding perceptions of aged body. First, the aged body as a system of signification that physicians examine bodies for indications that they mask the inner states of disorder. Second, the aged body as having a distinct pathology requiring medical therapy. Third, the aged body as dying. He argues that in pre-modern society, death was a mysterious external force while the science of the early nineteenth century re-conceptualized death as an internal phenomena of the body. Contemporary science is also engaged in re-conceptualizing death and old age (Vincent, 2007).

## Anti-ageing and Health

There are different views regarding anti-age. Post and Binstock (2004) said anti-aging interventions was a wide variety of ambitions and measures to slow, arrest, and reverse phenomena associated with aging. Mykytyn (2006) suggested that anti-aging medicine as a social movement and anti-aging's core mission is to herald and operationalize aging itself as treatable. Vincent (2007) suggested that anti-aging research refers exclusively to slowing, preventing, or reversing the aging process for the scientific community. In the medical and more reputable business community, anti-aging medicine means early detection, prevention, and reversal of age-related diseases. The wider business community views "anti-aging" as a valuable brand and a demonstrated way to increase sales. Broadly, and very charitably, it is looked at these varied definitions of anti-aging as meaning to look and feel younger in some way which has no bearing on how long you live or how healthy you actually are.

## Anti-aging and Health Care Prevention

In fact, anti-ageing is not an issue only about firming cream, anti-ageing facial treatments, cosmetic surgery, etc. It involves different aspects including beauty, medical, commercial, economy, and so on especially health care prevention.

Anti-aging means do something before ageing which is a preventative action. The aim is to achieve youth, beauty and health which can relieve the existing social ageing problems.

## Baby Boomers

Baby boomers are presently reaching middle age and beyond. They are retiring healthy, financially secure and with a desire to travel. Hong Kong Tourism Board (HKTB) executive director, Anthony Lau also said that

HKTB has identified the baby boomer segment as major target (Walker, 2009). University of Montreal demographer Jacques Legare said they have been independent their entire lives. They will not stop being self-reliant when they get old and sick. They have very few children and do not plan on counting on their progeny to look after them in their golden years. Legare also believes ageing baby boomers will radically change the health-care system and we will not put as much money in specialized medicine seeing as demand will mostly be for primary care (Hong Kong News Net, 2010).

Beginning with the post-World War II rise in consumption, boomers have been surrounded by commodities and advertising throughout their lives. In consequence, they are receptive to the calls of mass messaging. Part of boomers is still in the job market, many are still in or are back in the dating pool, and they have the money to spend on their wants. Recent advancements in technology provide an influx of new products and procedures to meet these demands. When members of this demographic are convinced that looking younger will provide them an edge at the office or interpersonally, they have the money and options to act on this desire and, thus strengthen the anti-aging market.

According to the U.S. Census this group represents 27.5 percent of the population, at approximately 77 million people (US Census Bureau, 2000). A demographic profile prepared by MetLife's Mature Market Institute reports the estimated annual spending power of baby boomers is 2.1 trillion dollars, and their annual average income is $56,000- $59,000 per year. If boomers are persuaded that they need to look younger, they are able to spend money on that need. The U.S. Census Bureau reports that baby boomers' 14.6 percent divorce rate is higher than prior generations. Also, the percentage of boomers who have never married is significantly higher than prior generations (MetLife, 2000). A greater number of baby boomers are dating in mid-life than in prior generations, and continue to be concerned with appearances and romantic attraction.

It ultimately suggests that as cosmetic technologies improve and access to such technologies widen, the anti-aging trend will grow stronger.

Further results are ageing health problem can be relieved while social economy can be stimulated.


## Age Discrimination

According to The American Society of Aesthetic Plastic Surgeons (ASAPS), nearly 6.9 million surgical and non-surgical cosmetic procedures were performed in 2002, an increase of 23 percent since 1997. Botox, a treatment that specifically targets age lines, ranked first among all surgical and non-surgical procedures in 2002. Based on 2001 statistics, non-surgical procedures with age defying benefits captured the top four procedures among all, with Botox ranking first, followed by chemical peel, collagen injection and microdermabrasion. Blepharoplasty, or cosmetic eyelid surgery, which provides the eyes with a younger, more alert appearance, was the top ranked facial surgery reported. It is also showed that concerns with aging are not exclusive to one gender. Though women made up approximately 88 percent of cosmetic procedures in 2001, the remaining 12 percent were undergone by men (ASAPS, 2003). An increasing cultural demand for anti-aging treatments among both genders occurred. Though men are more likely than women to say they want facial cosmetic procedures for work-related reasons, women cite this influence as well (American Academy of Facial Plastic and Reconstructive Surgery, 2002).

It is stressed that age discrimination maybe one of the work-related reasons for both genders seeking beauty treatment. Figure from previous chapter showing why Hong Kong women prefer cosmetic surgery gives support to it. Moreover, it is evidenced that older workers on average are more likely to be unemployed than younger ones on the labour market in Hong Kong. Unemployed workers aged above 45 tend to face a longer spell of unemployment, receive fewer job offers and expect lower future wages than the unemployed younger workers. Older employed workers may also be disadvantaged. The promotion and training opportunities available to older and younger employed workers are compared as well. It is found that older workers are less likely to be promoted or selected for training (Ho et al., 2000).

Census and Statistics Department (2009) revealed that 34.8% of the target population considered it acceptable to recruit employees of specific age ranges owing to the genuine practical need of certain occupations. Comparing with the situation of age discrimination in employment two years before the Survey, 37.7% of the target population thought that the situation had not changed, 21.7% considered that it had improved somewhat whilst 14.2% thought that it had worsened somewhat. The survey also showed that a significant portion of the target population, 34.8% as well as employers, 34.2% recognized that there was a genuine practical need for establishments in certain industries to recruit employees of a specified age range. It seems that some in the community considered it acceptable for establishments to do so. It is noted that the proportion of persons in the target group who perceived that age factor was the main reason for being rejected after job interview increased progressively with age, from 0.3% for persons aged 15-34 in the target group to 3.7% for persons aged 55 and over in the target group.

## DISCUSSION

It is situated that age discrimination within a broader system of age relations that intersects with other inequalities, defining old age as an unhealthy loss of gender identity (Calasanti, 2007). People would like to overcome ageing, keep them young and health to prevent such inequality. Anti-age is no longer appearance rejuvenation only. Both beauty and health should be the preventative tool and intervention to act the age related problems while society is what the government leads. It is understood that there are different needs of anti-ageing for different age groups. Three major groups can be separated to teach and support the different needs.

## Age at School: Health Education and Protection

Fundamental human biological cycle can be taught to every student. Growth, ageing and death should be understood. Enough nutrients are closely related for health and development while certain protection should be realized as well for beauty. For example, sun screener should be used for spot and skin cancer protection. It is suggested that the above information should be renewed and reinforced their importance according to the existing education.

## Age at Work: Health Protection and Promotion

Information is full of the world. Youth and middle age can get different information and product easily. With the basic beauty and health concept from the school, the most important in this stage is how to choose the suitable one and use correctly. It is observed that public chose and use in the wrong way have already harmed their health. In fact, majority possess healthy concept but not make themselves sufficient protection. Besides, it is encouraged public to start the plan earlier to stay young. It is also suggested that public health seminar and workshop of anti-stress can be promoted especially for the working adulthood to overcome stress which is the important factor to accelerate ageing (Horan et al., 2007).

## Age at Retirement: Health Promotion, Prevention and Protection

Anti-age at aged group should not be neglected. Health needs after retirement should be all the promotion, prevention and protection. One is protection of any healthy risks, second is prevention of nutrient loss, third is promotion of updated health information. Enough rich supplement, treatment, support and attitude of happiness to grow older should be promoted.

It is suggested that all different service departments like leisure and culture activities, communications and technology, education and training, employment, law, food and safety, health and medical services etc., should cooperate with beauty commercial and media and all should be lead by government for preventative anti-age actions. Accompany with the health protection scheme that is now encouraged by the Hong Kong government (FHB, 2010), public healthcare system is now reforming. The most important thing for long term public health care development is prevention and education. Anti-age is definitely an important issue of public health. Healthy supplements and beauty treatments can be discounted if public can attend certain exhibitions or seminars provided by the certificated age preventative health care intervention to support the health care system and encourage public to get the suitable and useful health information. To create a holistic health care system, good life-style and healthy social norm in Hong Kong, the medical expenses and social burden should be decreased in long term development. Healthy reputation can then be promoted worldwide to increase the competitiveness.

## CONCLUSION

Age related social problems like baby boomers and age discrimination of inequality are close related with public health. Anti-age science and technology can be applied on the beauty and health promotion to relieve the social burden and improve the social competitiveness. Anti-age is not only for people. Both beauty and health are also needed for each society. It is suggested that government should lead and coordinate with different departments for preventative anti-age actions earlier so that Hong Kong can keep young, energetic, beauty, and healthy image in the world.

# REFERENCES

American Academy of Facial Plastic and Reconstructive Surgery. (2002). Membership Survey: Trends in Facial Plastic Surgery. Retrieved December 12, 2010, from www.facemd.org

ASAPS. (2003). Retrieved December 12, 2010, from www.surgery.org

Bayer, K. (2004). *The Anti Aging Trend: Capitalism, Cosmetics and Mirroring the Spectacle.* Communication, Culture and Technology Program. Georgetown University.

Buss, D.M., & Schmitt, D.P. (1993). Sexual Strategies Theory: An evolutionary perspective on human mating. *Psychological Review, 100*,204-232.

Calasanti, T.M. (2007). Bodacious Berry, Potency Wood and the Aging Monster: Gender and Age Relations in Anti-Aging Ads. *Social Forces, 86*(1),335-355

CBSnews. (2003). Boomers seek fountain of youth. Retrieved December 13, 2010, from www.CBSnews.com.

Census and Statistics Department (2009). Thematic Household Survey Report No. 42: The Importance of Age Factor in Employment. Retrieved December 15, 2010, from http://www.legco.gov.hk/yr09-10/english/panels/mp/papers/mp1214cb2-523-5-e.pdf

Collins, M.A., & Zebrowitz, L.A. (1995). The contributions of appearance to occupational outcomes in civilian and military settings. *Journal of Applied Social Psychology, 25*,129-163.

Fetio, J. (2003). Image is Everything. *American Demographics*, 10-11.

Food and Health Bureau, FHB. (2010). Healthcare Reform Second Stage Public Consultation. Retrieved December 21, 2010, from http://www.myhealthmychoice.gov.hk/en/index.html

Foucault, M. (trans. A.M. Sheridan) (1973). *The Birth of the Clinic.* London: Routledge.

Haberer, J. (2010). *In search of beauty.* GRIN Publishing.

Hoareau, L., & DaSilva, E.J. (1999). Medicinal plants: a re-emerging health aid. *Plant Biotechnology, 2*(2).

Ho, L.S., Wei, X.D., & Voon, J.P. (2000). Are Older Workers Disadvantaged in the Hong Kong Labour Market? *Asian Economic Journal, 14*(3),283-300.

Hong Kong News Net. (2010). Baby boomers ageing to be self-reliant. Retrieved December 20, 2010, from http://www.hongkongnews. net/story/628106

Horan, M.A., Barton, R.N., & Lithgow, G.J. (2007). Aging and Stress, Biology of. *Encyclopedia of Stress* (2nd edition, 102-107).

Joshi, D.K. (2006). Orissa Review: Health Care Practices of Tribals. Retrieved December 12, 2010, from http://www.orissa.gov.in/e-magazine/Orissareview/dec-2006/engpdf/dec.pdf#page=55

Katz, S. (1996). *Disciplining Old Age: The Formation of Gerontological Knowledge*. London: University Press of Virginia.

MetLife. (2000). US Census Bureau, 2000, Demographic Profile, American Baby Boomers. Retrieved December 20, 2010, from www. metlife.com.

Mykytyn, C.E. (2006). Anti-aging medicine: A patient/ practioner movement to redefine aging. *Social Science and Medicine, 62*,643-653.

Post, S.G., & Binstock, R.H. (2004) *The Fountain of Youth: Cultural, Scientific, and Ethical Perspectives on a Biomedical Goal*. Oxford: Oxford University Press.

Shostak, S. (2002) *Becoming Immortal: Combining Cloning and Stem-cell Therapy*. Albany: State University of New York Press.

US Census Bureau. (2000). Factifinder, Age groups and sex: 2000. Retrieved from December 20, 2010, from www.census.gov.

Vincent, J.A. (2007). Science and imagery in the 'war on old age'. *Ageing and Society*, 27,941-961.

Walker, K. (2009). Hong Kong Tourism targets Boomers. Retrieved December 20, 2010, from http://silvergroup.asia/blog/Hong-Kong-Tourism-targets-Boomers.php

# ABOUT THE AUTHOR

Zenobia C. Y. Chan. Assistant Professor, School of Nursing, The Hong Kong Polytechnic University. Phone: 852-2766 6426; Email: hszchan@ inet.polyu.edu.hk; zehippo@yahoo.com

Zenobia Chan is an assistant professor of the School of Nursing, at the Hong Kong Polytechnic University. She received her Bachelor's Degree in Nursing, and her Master's Degrees in Primary Health Care and Christian Studies in 1999 and 2008 respectively. She obtained a Doctoral Degree in Social Welfare from The Chinese University of Hong Kong in 2003. Zenobia loves writing for both its therapeutic and communicative uses. She has written for a wide range of academic journals and has contributed five English books (such as Silenced Women Published by the Nova Science Publishers) and two Chinese books. She has published papers related to nursing, family studies, counseling, mental health, medical education, social work, qualitative research and poetry. In hopes of contributing to healthcare research, Zenobia serves as an editorial member and a reviewer of referred journals.

# INDEX

## E

## D

**F**

**G**

## T